Restoring Primary Care

The authors dedicate this book to their wives,
Linda and Deborah, to the patients whose stories
motivate us to work to improve primary care, and
to the colleagues who inspire our hope
and provide a way forward.

Restoring Primary Care

REFRAMING RELATIONSHIPS AND REDESIGNING PRACTICE

ANTON J KUZEL

MD, MHPE
Department of Family Medicine
Virginia Commonwealth University

and

JOHN D ENGEL

PhD
Institute for Professionalism Inquiry
Summa Health System
Department of Behavioral Sciences
Northeastern Ohio Universities College of Medicine

Foreword by
DAVID LOXTERKAMP

MD

Afterword by
WILLIAM L MILLER

MD, MA

Radcliffe Publishing
Oxford • New York

Radcliffe Publishing Ltd
18 Marcham Road
Abingdon
Oxon OX14 1AA
United Kingdom

www.radcliffepublishing.com

Electronic catalogue and worldwide online ordering facility.

British Library Cataloguing in Publication Data

A catalogue record for this book is available from the British Library.

ISBN-13: 978 184619 382 8

The paper used for the text pages of this book
is FSC certified. FSC® (The Forest Stewardship
Council®) is an international network to promote
responsible management of the world's forests.

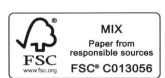

Typeset by Pindar NZ, Auckland, New Zealand
Printed and bound by TJI Digital, Padstow, Cornwall, UK

Contents

Foreword

THE REFLECTIVE PRACTITIONER AND THE GOALS OF MEDICINE

When Tony Kuzel and John Engel asked me to write the Foreword to their book, they suggested that I "speak to what is needed to reinvigorate primary care from the perspective of the reflective practitioner." It had been almost 20 years since I first heard that phrase, while on sabbatical at the University of California, San Francisco, and its memory excited me. The reformation of primary care is often seen as a systems problem—how to get payers to pay for it, students to study it, and coordinated teams to tackle it. Little attention is afforded to the select few professionals who can actually steer us there. I am not talking about visionaries, educators, or policy-makers, but primary care leaders in patient care. What motivates them? What discourages them? What prepares them for the hard but gratifying work of shared leadership? What keeps them from burning out?

In their book, Drs Kuzel and Engel offer a clear, practical, and evidence-based guide for the transformation of primary care practice. It is intended for those unwilling to sit on their hands until the conditions are right. Their program, like many, will achieve the end product of an NCQA (National Committee for Quality Assurance) certified patient-centered medical house. But they are reaching for something more. They challenge us to make it a home and to think carefully about who will live there.

Let me begin the conversation. First, I'll describe my own experience with home construction over the last quarter century. Next, I'll revisit Donald Schon's classic text, *The Reflective Practitioner: how professionals think in action.*[1] And lastly, I'll talk about leadership and its elusive shadow, offering another way to consider vision, strength, and the goals of medicine.

In January of 2010, my practice joined the Maine Patient Centered Medical Home Pilot. Over the next three years, we expect to receive a monthly payment for every patient who is an active enrollee in the state Medicaid program plus three private insurance companies. The 10% boost in annual revenues will allow us to experiment with office reconfiguration, the addition of ancillary staff, and an opportunity to participate in a network of physicians and practices who are enthusiastically embracing practice reform. It has taken us 25 years to get to this point. Milestones include:

1992	Becoming a rural health center
1994	Choosing our first electronic medical record (EMR) system
2004	Prescribing Suboxone for opioid addicts
2005	Building a new office
2006	Implementing our second EMR; beginning the National Demonstration Project
2007	Offering a patient portal
2008	Adjusting to open scheduling
2009	Recruiting two young family physicians and a physician's assistant.

Inexplicably, one step leads to another. Becoming a rural health center doubled our salaries overnight, largely by paying us for the cost of treating Medicaid patients. Our first electronic medical record taught us what to look for in the next. Office-based treatment of opioid dependence provided our first exposure to population management, mental health care, and working with a systems approach. The National Demonstration Project nudged us to make two simple changes in our practice that dramatically transformed it: open scheduling (which allows same-day access to the provider) and a patient portal (which allows instant access to the entire medical record and greater accountability, partnering, and email communication). Finally, successful recruitment has given us hope for the future, the ability to extend office hours, and the opportunity to build the kind of practice we always imagined.

In their "Ten steps to a patient-centered medical home" (Chapter 6), Kuzel and Engel are squarely on target. They describe the key interlocking pieces of a congruent whole, the assembly of which takes imagination, perseverance, and bit of luck.

In 1984, my wife and I moved to Belfast, Maine. Shortly thereafter, I formed a partnership with Tim Hughes, a family doctor who shared my sense of humor, love of stories, and practice philosophy. But six years of caring for the infirm, pregnant, critically ill, homebound, poor and marginalized took their toll. We both needed a break. While I "held the fort," Tim spent a year in Costa Rica establishing a new family medicine residency program; I left the following year for the West Coast.

It was around this time that men with AIDS were returning to Waldo County, often to reconcile with their families, always to die. HIV was unknown during my residency, and in the first years of practice it was barely understood or adequately treated. As I looked around for fellowship sites, San Francisco seemed a logical location. I was accepted at the Family and Community Medicine Fellowship Program at San Francisco General Hospital, then directed by Dr Peter Sommers. It was during his seminars that we read Donald Schon's groundbreaking work. I felt then, and still believe, that this professor of urban studies and education at Massachusetts Institute of Technology (MIT) thoroughly understood how accomplished family physicians worked, and where the discipline must lead the transformation of primary care.

In his book, Schon was critical of what he saw as the dominant pattern of professional thinking, something he called *technical rationality*. In this mindset, practice is a problem-solving activity undertaken by professionals who alone decide which problems are appropriate, how they should be treated, and what to do with conflicting data. When raw data does not conform to the canon of fixable problems, the expert discards it. And where people are at "fault," they are labeled as outliers, malingerers, or neurotics.

Schon agreed that emergencies and routines require a precise and methodical approach. But he was more interested in the moment before action, when professionals frame their experience as recognizable problems, or later, when these problems do not respond in the expected way. He described *reflection-in-action* as the ability of a professional to adjust to surprise, frustration, or failure, and to make corrections in understanding or technique while the outcome is still in question.[1] The work of primary care always begins by "setting" or framing the problem. Is it a medical problem? Does the patient want or need it fixed? Is treatment failure the result of a misdiagnosis, the need for more time, or an incomplete grasp of the setting?

For Schon, the reflective practitioner was someone who welcomed surprise. Reward came not from achieving a certain level of proficiency in treating familiar problems, but from a sense of discovery in the strangeness, instability, uncertainty, and conflicting values of the problem at hand. Rather than working safely in pre-existing categories, he joined the patient in a shared, intuitive, and largely creative process. The setting for that process was a relationship where the doctor focuses on the quality of a life, using his own as a reference point.

The reflective practitioner "gives up the rewards of unquestioned authority, the freedom to practice without challenge to his competence, the comfort of relative invulnerability, the gratifications of deference. The new satisfactions open to him are largely those of discovery—about the meanings of his advice to clients, about his knowledge-in-practice, and about himself."[1]

Kurt, a 24-year-old on state assistance, is enrolled in our office-based treatment program for opioid dependence. He faithfully sees an addiction counselor every week and a medical provider every other week. His daily dose of Suboxone (which contains buprenorphine, a partial opioid agonist) is only 8 mg a day. He smokes cigarettes, but doesn't drink alcohol, and his urine drug screens have always been "clean." Kurt also takes medication and receives a disability pension for Bipolar disease.

Though he has been coming to the office for six months, this is only the second time we've met. I learn that he is neither employed nor in school. He dropped out of high school and expresses no interest in earning a GED. He currently lives with his father and watches television in his room all day. He has a girlfriend who works two seasonal jobs for minimum wage. And though they have lived together for the past four years, he has no plans to marry or have children.

He returns today for a refill of his Suboxone and to discuss smoking cessation. At last visit, he set a quit date and began wearing a nicotine patch. But after three days, he resumed smoking, stating that it was "just too hard."

> "What are you willing to work on?" I inquire.
> Kurt turns with a puzzled look. "Nothing, I guess. I'm just lazy, and always have been."

I am curious, annoyed, and baffled by his lack of spark, but also by his honesty. He tells me that he and his therapist mostly watch videos about addiction. They do not discuss "plans," a topic that troubles him, he admits, largely because it troubles his father and girlfriend.

So what is the doctor to do? Am I "treating" his addiction or "enabling" his laziness and indecision—or both? Should I continue to prescribe Suboxone because it is working? Should he stay in counseling because he attends it regularly? Should I urge him to see a therapist who will challenge his self-diagnosis of laziness, or offer a psychiatric referral to revisit his label of Bipolar disease? Should I taper him off Suboxone if he is unwilling to work on anything in life, or continue it because he has chronic opioid dependence (which, of course, my prescription maintains)?

By asking, "Is laziness a problem?" have I over-reached my professional bounds or imposed my own values? Is it equally lazy—even unethical—for health professionals to ignore the biopsychosocial determinants of disease and maintain our patients in dependent relationships? What are the goals of medicine?

This is the question increasingly asked as our focus becomes patient-centered. Because primary care physicians (PCPs) form relationships with their patients, certain questions are obvious and relevant: "Why is the patient here today? What is the source of his unhappiness? Can I help him identify or resolve it, whatever it is?"

The proponents of motivational interviewing (MI)—first described by William Miller and Stephen Rollnick—encourage and prepare us to be catalysts for change in the troubled lives of our patients. They emphasize that MI is less "technique" than conversation, more an invitation for the patient to work through his ambivalence than a contest for change.[2] The patient's readiness matters, but so does the doctor's demonstrated investment and confidence in the patient's future.

Having passed a quarter-century of caring for patients, I am aware and confident of my habits in the exam room. The most effective are these:

➤ Let patients know you are glad to see them.
➤ Meet their eyes, as it expresses your concern and reveals what words cannot.
➤ Touch them, especially where they are diseased. This is the physical expression of our intent to provide a sense of connection and approval.
➤ Only give advice that addresses their goals.
➤ And make sure they understand what is wrong, when they'll be better, and what to do if they're not.

John Scott and others have described healing environments or settings that rely upon the sensitivity, skill, and contribution of each member. Almost 30 years ago, Schon provided his own vision of such a place:

> A reflective institution must place a high priority on flexible procedures, differentiated responses, qualitative appreciation of complex processes, and decentralized responsibility for judgment and action. In contrast to the normal bureaucratic emphasis on technical rationality, a reflective institution must make a place for attention to conflicting values and purposes.[1]

In the section, "Essentials for the journey" from Chapter 6, Kuzel and Engel also focus on the health care team. They ask why certain teams—and the practices they serve—work better than others. Borrowing from Tony Ghaye and his book, *Developing the Reflective Healthcare Team*, they look to the qualities of team members. Leaders emerge who exhibit a kind of "quiet leadership" that seeks to change their own behavior before requiring it of others; fosters a culture of questioning and problem solving; puts team goals before personal agenda; allows decisions to be made at the level where they most directly applied; and cultivates an "emotional awareness" that informs decision making.[3] This kind of leadership is seen less easily in the attributes of a single provider than through the influence cast upon the team and its goals.

In our experience with practice innovation, curiosity has always been the driving force, pushing us to weigh, compare, question, and challenge our current practices against the deficiencies we live with and toward an elusive "ideal." Curiosity is tempered by the need for tolerance, understanding that not everyone may need to change, or change to the same degree, or change at the same pace. Humility reminds us of our limitations and the need for others' insights. Transparency is a sign of self-confidence; it promotes mutual respect and a sense of inclusion. We have come to regard change itself as a positive value, preferring it to the familiar, easy, and predictable. Lastly, struggle to place greater value on relationships than the "bottom line," knowing how easily the sense of human connection can be pinched by the pressures of efficiency, quantification, and financial reward.

I am not sure that my practice succeeds as a reflective or healing environment. Such attention takes time. It distracts from the business at hand. It leads to disappointing results based on conventional measures of quality. It requires hard work and commands an ever higher bar. But it is, I believe, what our patients need and deserve as we engage them in extended, committed relationships, remaining curious and questioning about the causes of illness and means to health. There are others who can apply protocols more consistently, automatically, and routinely than a family doctor, including computers and technicians. This is not where our skills are required. Rather, it seems to me, our role lies in uncovering the unique elements inside a patient's concern, at this moment in time, impeding their pursuit of health as they define it.

Why don't more doctors improve the health of their practices? Why can't we make them responsive, effective, and joyous places to work? What Ira Glass, host of National Public Radio's *This American Life*, recently said about writing applies equally to the practice of medicine: "It's like a law of nature, a law of aerodynamics, that anything that's written or anything that's created wants to be mediocre. The natural state of all writing is mediocrity. It's all tending toward mediocrity in the same way that all atoms are sort of dissipating out toward the expanse of the universe. [. . .] So what it takes to make anything more than mediocre is such an act of will."[4] That act requires a spark, something that needs fuel to flame and friendship to spread and shelter it. Good medicine requires our attention to deeply buried needs and injuries. It is simple and universal and achievable in every encounter. By offering it to others, it is returned to us in full. It is the work of the reflective practitioner, the yeast of a healing environment, and the fundamental goal of all medicine. It stems from the awareness that the doctor and patient share a similar need: to take responsibility for their own happiness. The most satisfying and effective way to learn this is through a nurturing relationship wherein what the doctor offers—often, all we offer—is conversation, friendship, and hope.

David Loxterkamp, MD
Belfast, Maine
September 2010

REFERENCES

1 Schon D. *The Reflective Practitioner: how professionals think in action.* New York, NY: Basic Books; 1983. pp. 229, 338.

2 Miller WR, Rollnick S. *Motivational Interviewing: preparing people for change.* 2nd ed. New York, NY: Guilford Press; 2002.

3 Ghaye T. *Developing the Reflective Healthcare Team.* Malden, MA: Wiley-Blackwell; 2006.

4 Glass I. Quoted in Keillor G. *The Writer's Almanac;* March 3, 2010. Available at: http:// writersalmanac.publicradio.org/index.php?date=2010/03/03 (accessed March 30, 2010).

Preface

This book represents a connecting of dots—linking prior studies we and others have done on patient safety with the current movement on practice redesign in primary care. As we reflected on the avoidable problems and harms in the primary care experiences of patients in Virginia and Ohio with whom we spoke several years ago, we realized that many of the primary care redesign strategies (advocated most notably by the Institute for Healthcare Improvement) would directly address those problems and likely lead to safer, more effective care for patients. They would also foster a relationship-centered primary care environment that, in our view, is the real point of the so-called patient-centered medical home.

We are also alarmed by the enormous shift away from primary care in the US that has occurred over the past 15–20 years, which is due in part to cultural factors in the US and in the places where most doctors train, but mostly due to the bizarre way in which care is financed (and therefore incentivized) in the US. There is no systematic push to improve the health of patients or populations, but rather enormous incentives to perform tests and treatments on people, often with little or no evidence of benefit. We hear and support the calls for reforming the financing of health care in the US so as to reduce or eliminate the perverse incentives, but the recently passed health care reform act, while admittedly the most significant change in health care policy in the US since the establishment of Medicare and Medicaid in 1965, does little to change incentives (except through pilot projects). While it provides new coverage for about 30 million US citizens, it doesn't do much to also ensure that they will have access to primary health care.

The reason for this partial achievement is, in our view, because a system that focused on population care and that is based in primary care would create dramatic shifts in funding away from the entities and individuals who now profit greatly from the current arrangements. Knowing that it will likely be 10 or 20 years before the rest of reform is passed (the politics are daunting), we feel a sense of urgency to help create change *now*, and we look for strategies to improve existing primary care practices that don't depend upon further fundamental reforms, that are easily understood by the average primary care practice team, and that are drawn from actual practices, i.e. that have been tested and found useful.

We finally wanted to suggest a sequence of successful strategies—not our ideas, but perhaps a novel way of once again connecting the dots—that would start with improving the financial well-being of practices. While the self-actualization of practices is an important end to have in mind, the work of American psychologist Abraham Maslow, who conceptualized a pyramidal hierarchy of five fundamental human motivational needs (from satisfying basic and physiological needs to self-actualization), suggests that practice finances—the analogue of food, clothing, and shelter—should receive first attention. We hear so many people who have studied practice transformation say that it is difficult, that it takes a long time, and that it requires starting with practice culture and leadership. While there is merit in these perspectives, we are concerned that this might feel like jumping to self-actualization. We worry that this view doesn't offer a ready way to engage the typical practice whose clinicians and staff feel overworked, underappreciated, and underpaid. Therefore, we choose in this book to offer instead a sequence of steps that can *result* in a healthier office culture, enlightened leadership, and practice self-actualization. We see these ends as inherent in the aspirations of most people who want to deliver primary care—they are drawn to the specialty because of a love of longitudinal, relationship-based care. Might not practices that use strategies to improve their efficiency and effectiveness also be places in which the better angels of the clinicians and staff can re-emerge?

We begin in Chapter 1 by reviewing a study we published a few years back in which we asked patients served by family physicians, general internists, and general pediatricians in Virginia and Ohio to tell us their stories of avoidable problems and harms they or their loved ones had experienced during their care. We continue in Chapter 2 with a series of narratives based on our interviews that portray some of the most common or most compelling themes. We offer in Chapter 3 a way of reconceptualizing so-called patient-centered care as relationship-centered care, a move very consistent with the ethics and power of team care. Chapter 4 describes the current movement in the US towards patient-centered and relationship-centered care, and Chapter 5 offers a sample of stories of success, many of which informed the model that follows in Chapter 6. This 10-step model is meant to be a practical prescription for distressed primary care practices. We include as appendices a wonderful practice self-assessment tool developed by John Wasson and others at Dartmouth, as well as a "readers theater" that health professional educators may use to vividly illustrate what ails overburdened primary care practices in the US.

This book is for those dedicated clinicians, staff, and administrators who wonder where the joy of primary care has gone, and how to reclaim it in the midst of polarized politics and the resistance to change from those who are financially benefiting most from our hugely expensive, ineffective health care system. It is not meant to be a capitulation to those forces, but rather a means to re-moralize (in the sense of moral *and* morale) the dedicated teams doing their best to provide primary care to their patients. We want to help them make their work a little easier, and hope that a renewal of energy and effect will not enable the continued dysfunctions of our system of care and financing, but rather enable the rejuvenated practices to serve as examples of what our system of care and financing must celebrate and sustain. Perhaps with a little more emotional reserve, some of these practices can become more engaged in advocacy for continuing reform—they will certainly have the moral authority to be a powerful voice for change. We offer this book with the humble wish that its messages and suggestions help achieve these ends.

Anton J Kuzel, Richmond, Virginia
John D Engel, Surry, Maine
September 2010

About the authors

Anton J Kuzel, MD, MHPE, is Harris-Mayo Professor and Chair of Family Medicine at Virginia Commonwealth University, Richmond, Virginia. His Masters in Health Professions Education was completed at the Center for Educational Development, University of Illinois at the Medical Center, Chicago, where John Engel, PhD, served as his principal advisor and introduced him to qualitative research traditions, including critical social science. Since then, he has worked both as a qualitative methodologist and researcher, most recently in the area of medical errors in primary care and in barriers to delivery of preventive health services. He is also actively engaged with academic and professional organizations to promote the redesign of primary care at the local and regional level.

John D Engel, PhD, a social scientist, is Scientific Director of the Institute for Professionalism Inquiry, Summa Health System, and Professor Emeritus of Behavioral Science at the Northeastern Ohio Universities College of Medicine. His research interests are the philosophy of social science inquiry, qualitative methodology, narrative health care, and integrating humanities and social sciences with health professions education and practice and care of the dying. John served as founding associate editor for *Qualitative Health Research* and edited the methodology section of that journal. He has been a member of the Editorial Board of *Evaluation and the Health Professions* since its inception. He has published extensively in his areas of interest, and is currently engaged in conducting a longitudinal study of professional development as well as a participatory action project on the impact of narrative practice in a department of family medicine.

Acknowledgments

The authors wish to thank the co-investigators who helped field and publish the study on patient reports of medical errors that appears in the first chapter—Steven Woolf, Valerie Gilchrist, Thomas LaVeist, Charles Vincent, and Richard Frankel. They also thank Barbara Wright, research librarian at Virginia Commonwealth University, who provided invaluable assistance with finding key citations. We greatly appreciate the help of Clarisse Harton who assisted in the final production of the manuscript. Finally, we thank the editors of Radcliffe Publishing, Michael Hawkes and Gillian Nineham, who not only improved the finished manuscript, but who provided us the opportunity to share stories of suffering and of hope, and practical strategies for revitalizing primary care in the US.

Anton J Kuzel, Richmond, Virginia
John D Engel, Surry, Maine
September 2010

CHAPTER 1

Avoidable problems and harms in primary care

PROLOGUE

The patient safety movement in the US got a political shot in the arm in 1999 with the publication of *To Err is Human*, a work produced by the Institute of Medicine (IOM) within the National Academies of Science that concluded that as many as 98 000 people died in US hospitals every year from avoidable causes.[1] This led to a public outcry and Congressional hearings that, in turn, led Congress to mandate that the Agency for Healthcare Research and Quality (AHRQ) create and field a program of study to identify the causes of avoidable harms in US health care, particularly in hospital settings, and to identify and disseminate strategies to mitigate those contributing factors.

Shortly after the IOM report was released, one of my (AK) colleagues in the Department of Family Medicine at Virginia Commonwealth University, Steven Woolf, approached me at a faculty meeting and shared with me several concerns he had about the report. First, he wasn't sure that the report was entirely clear about what constituted a medical error; second, the cited studies were all based in hospital settings, and we both knew that the vast majority of health care in the US and elsewhere occurred in ambulatory settings; and, third, the perspectives reported on were those of health care professionals, with no specific attention to the views of patients. He found all of this troubling, and asked if I would be interested in creating a grant proposal to address these concerns in some way. I quickly agreed, and brought in John Engel and several other collaborators to create a proposal to address these concerns. We responded to the first Request for Applications (RFA) from the AHRQ on patient safety, and were fortunate to be funded for the work we proposed.* Our study's aims, design, and findings were published in the *Annals of Family Medicine* in 2004,[2] and are reproduced at

---

* An explanation of the process for writing a qualitative research proposal for this kind of work may be found in an article we published in *Qualitative Health Research*.[3]

the close of this chapter with the permission of the publisher. We continue with a representation of our thoughts about our findings at the time of publication, and summarize the work about patient and provider perspectives about medical errors in primary care that have been published in the ensuing years.

DISCUSSION

This study found that the medical errors related by patients in our sample are more likely to involve the breakdowns in the clinician–patient relationship and the access to clinicians than the technical errors that are the focus of current patient safety initiatives. The patients we interviewed spoke more about insensitivity and miscommunication than, for example, receiving the wrong drug prescription.

This perspective contrasts sharply with what recent research shows family physicians report. Physician reports are dominated by breakdowns in information transfer and ultimate treatment errors,[4,5] whereas our results suggest that patients cite problems of access and relationship, which are dominated by psychological injuries. Our findings resonate with others who have urged giving more attention to patient perspectives of medical errors[6] and with recent surveys suggesting that the public and the medical community view patient safety through different lenses.[7–10]

Our study has a number of potential limitations. First, the interview subjects were self-selected, and their personal experiences might not be representative of the general primary care population. Second, the respondents were asked to recall problematic incidents from their entire past experience, so their reports are likely to be the most recent or the most memorable incidents. Third, the modest sample size further limits the generalizability of our findings. Fourth, the proportions we report are sensitive to our typology and the validity of our denominators, which others might contest.

Finally, our report includes as errors a broad range of problematic experiences that might fall outside others' sense of the term. As stated earlier, we conceive of errors as all forms of improper, delayed, or omitted care that unnecessarily injures patients by either worsening health outcomes or causing physical or emotional distress. We defend the inclusion of emotional distress as a legitimate, preventable harm—mistakes that cause patients to be frightened or humiliated are just as important as those that cause physical distress—but including emotional distress creates an indistinct boundary between medical errors and patient dissatisfaction. The frustration that patients experience with, for example, long appointment delays may be relevant to some and trivial to others. We recognize this difficulty, but we reasoned that it was preferable to use liberal boundaries to obtain a complete picture of what patients dislike about their care and to allow others to judge what subset of those problems they choose to label as errors. Further, we think it unwise to ignore the frustrating and dehumanizing experiences that erode a relationship which has caring as its imperative. One can also argue that whether the label of errors applies may be less important than recognizing the preventable harms associated with primary health care.

Layde *et al.*[6] remind us that injury prevention is the goal of quality improvement. The stories we solicited reverberated with recurring and troubling themes: You cannot get a human being on the telephone, and you cannot get an appointment. When you do have an appointment, you wait an excessive time before seeing the doctor, who is in a hurry, does not seem to care, and provides inadequate explanation and education. There were several stories of perceived racism. The interviews suggest a variety of experiences that can act to potentiate harmful outcomes and that may lead to a common final pathway for dissatisfaction and poor-quality care. Our study respondents received emotional injury in many ways, but each event had the potential to weaken the patient's relationship with the clinician and culminate in loss of trust in the health care system. This outcome carries a potentially large public health burden given the principle that small disturbances in a large number of cases create a large population effect.

These narratives also underscore that deficiencies in every critical feature of the system—accessibility, timeliness, patient-centeredness, effectiveness, efficiency and safety[11]—are capable of producing harm. As suggested recently by Lee,[12] rather than focus on errors or any other particular segment in isolation, the totality warrants simultaneous attention. Illustrating a theme of *To Err is Human*,[1] these stories of errors and harms speak to system design flaws that are amenable to analysis and change.[13,14] Some changes in primary care systems stimulated by consortia such as the Institute for Healthcare Improvement[15] (e.g. open-access scheduling,[16] electronic medical records[17]) might ameliorate some of the errors patients report, but they do not directly address the rushed, dehumanizing health care experiences that pervade our narratives. This aspect of our findings resonates with recent survey studies that show a decline in patient ratings of the quality of their interactions with their PCPs.[18,19]

The current emphasis by the American Association of Medical Colleges (AAMC) on professionalism in medical education[20] and its enforcement of 80-hour resident workweeks[21] are important efforts, but what of the persistent and considerable pressures on faculty and residents for clinical productivity? Will primary care clinicians, faced with increasing overhead from regulatory requirements and malpractice costs, be able, even if willing, to deliver patient-centered care? Will they be able to afford the quantity and quality of staff, and spend sufficient time with their patients? We believe it will require major reforms in medical education, in the financing of health care, and in the manner in which we deal with injuries associated with health care to alter the substrate for breakdowns in relationships with clinicians.

To read or post commentaries in response to this article, see it online at www.annfammed.org/cgi/content/full/2/4/333.

Funding support: This project was supported by grant number: U18HS11117–01 from the AHRQ.

AFTER OUR STUDY

There have been many other studies about patient safety in ambulatory primary care settings since the time of our work. Elder *et al.* surveyed Cincinnati family physicians to ascertain what kinds of errors they perceived in their offices, and with what relative frequency. Their survey tool was structured around several error categories: diagnosis (wrong, delayed, or missed), management and treatment (inappropriate, delayed, omitted, or procedural complication), physicians and staff (judgment, skill, communication, rushed, interrupted), chart elements (missing, misplaced, or incorrect), office administration (charts, forms, personnel, reminder systems), and investigations and flow (incorrect or delayed investigations, problems with referrals, triage, or phone messages). Responders identified errors or preventable adverse events in fully 24% of office visits, with most of these being in the category of office administration.[22] Phillips *et al.* reviewed malpractice claims against PCPs in the US and found that the majority of cases occurred in the outpatient setting and typically involved failure to diagnose or delay in diagnosis, particularly conditions such as ischemic heart disease, various cancers, and appendicitis.[23] One of us (AK) participated in an international study of physician reports of errors in primary care,[4] and found that the majority of reports from US PCPs could be understood as a chain or cascade of errors. Most of these were mistakes in treatment or diagnosis, but communication breakdowns were involved in 80% of the reports. Although psychological harms to patients were reported in only 17% of cases, we believed we could confidently infer psychological harm in nearly 70% of the reports.[24] Similar patterns were found in the other participating countries.[5,25] Other studies focused on problems with tracking, responding to, and communicating test results,[26-30] avoidable problems associated with prescription drugs,[31,32] missing clinical information,[33,34] "hand-offs" (e.g. transfers from hospital care back to primary care),[35] and new problems unique to the use of electronic medical records.[36] Family physicians in the US do not have a shared working definition of what constitutes an error, with the vast majority agreeing that ordering the wrong test or not following up on abnormal test results constituted an error, but only half seeing the breaking of a vial of blood and the resulting need for repeat venipuncture as an error.[37] Bearing this lack of consensus in mind, it is nonetheless interesting that an Australian study of general practitioners suggests that an error occurs between one and two times for every 1000 patients seen,[38] and a similar rate was found in a survey of patients in the Midwestern US.[39] Confidential reports by general practitioners in the UK suggest that mistakes in situation assessment and response were the most common sorts of errors, and that these were in turn attributed to excessive task demands and to fragmented care processes.[40]

Studies that, like our own, focused on patient perceptions and experiences of medical error in primary care settings, revealed themes consistent with those we found. A focus group study of patients from urban locales in the Midwest US emphasized problems with access to care, long waits in the office, poor listening skills of physicians, technical errors, and medication errors.[41] A survey of about 2000 patients cared for in primary care clinics in Minnesota asked if patients had experienced a wrong diagnosis, treatment, prescription, procedure, or some other form of medical error during their last visit to their PCPs. Physician and nurse reviewers in this study went back to the medical record and re-categorized nearly half of the reports as "misunderstandings" when it appeared to them that the patient had not felt heard or responded to in the way he or she desired. Another 20% seemed to reflect on the behavior of non-physician personnel at the site of care, including excessive waiting times, rudeness, or inadequate explanations.[39] A survey of members of rural and frontier communities in the western US again provided evidence of conventionally defined medical errors, including diagnostic delays, missed diagnoses, and medication errors. The open-ended responses also contained some themes reminiscent of our study, including violations of trust, unmet expectations between patients and clinicians, and unacceptable deportment of health care professionals.[42] A study in the Netherlands that compared various identification strategies found that patients were more likely to report avoidable problems in their care and that these included breach of confidentiality, lack of respect by the physician, delay in diagnosis, wrong medication prescribed, wrong advice, or errors in appointment scheduling.[43] Wasson *et al.* demonstrated that patients will report errors via the internet and that patients with higher illness burden were far more likely to report problems with their care.[44] Although there may be disagreement about what constitutes an error, there is evidence to suggest that patients who experience "service quality deficiencies" are also more likely to report a medical error, more narrowly defined.[39,45] Our two studies and the others we reviewed demonstrate that physicians and patients do not have consensus on what constitutes a medical error, and that many of the problems seen by one group are invisible to the other group.

What constitutes a medical error? We want to reiterate a key position we take in the discussion section of the paper: "[W]e conceive of errors as all forms of improper, delayed, or omitted care that unnecessarily injures patients by either worsening health outcomes or causing physical or emotional distress." We firmly believe that these sorts of preventable harms are important to address and avoid. As succinctly put by James Bagian, the Chief Patient Safety Officer for the Veterans Affairs Health System, it's all about harm reduction.[46] Can't we think of some of these as "relationship mistakes?" Don't these sorts of preventable problems diminish our ability to engage in empathic relationships with our patients? By empathic relationship, we have in mind curiosity and emotional resonance[47]—"a housecall from one human spirit to another."[48] Empathy is critical for relationship-centered and narrative health care because it helps people tolerate intolerable feelings; it helps people believe the future might not be as bad as they think; and it helps people regain agency and self-efficacy.[47,49] Patients want empathy, and physicians benefit as well! Empathic relationships have been associated with:

➤ more thorough diagnoses[50]
➤ greater effectiveness[51–53]
➤ less physician burnout[54]
➤ little or no extra time expended.[55]

Furthermore, there is evidence that when patients are involved in decision-making and treated with dignity, that both features independently contribute to patient satisfaction and adherence to treatment.[56]

What's at stake? Death by a thousand cuts—the accumulation of small insults and injuries that erodes trust and destroys one of the most important relationships in our lives—the one we have with our primary care clinician.

How did primary care in the US get to be in such a sorry state? Many factors have surely contributed, but we believe some of the major issues include the following:

➤ Financing of health care that incentivizes the testing and treatment of individuals rather than maintaining the health of a population.
➤ No mechanism for an effective national health care workforce plan, allowing "market forces" to determine the mix and distribution of physicians, with only modest efforts to impact the supply and distribution.
➤ A Medicare payment advisory board comprised almost entirely of

procedural subspecialists which has emphasized payments for procedures over cognitively based care.

➤ A growing gap in incomes between PCPs and subspecialists—in the late 1980s, PCPs made about 80% of the average income of subspecialists, and now they make approximately half of a subspecialist's income. Primary care income has actually fallen over the past decade when corrected for inflation.

➤ Growing administrative oversight by payers and the resulting burdens that fall disproportionately on PCPs, who have had to hire extra staff just to keep up with the complexities of the polyglot of payers and rules for payment for services.

➤ A basic model for primary care delivery that was developed over 100 years ago when acute care medicine was the dominant form of primary care.

➤ A degradation in the primary care workforce as US medical students flock to the "ROAD to success" specialties (i.e. Radiology, Ophthalmology, Anesthesiology, Dermatology), resulting in pressure on existing PCPs to carry larger panels of patients than they are currently equipped to handle.

➤ PCPs leaving front-line service positions relatively early in their careers as a result of professional burnout, further exacerbating the pressures on those that remain.

What has resulted is what too often can be called "hamster wheel medicine"[57] in which primary care clinicians rush through visits and feel overwhelmed by ever-increasing administrative burdens and overhead costs with no accompanying increase in payments for their professional services. This has led to disillusionment and a loss of morale and meaning for such clinicians, and it is our belief that this environment was the backdrop for many of the patient stories in our study. Moreover, many primary care clinicians feel they are in a classic catch-22 scenario: a no-win situation with no way to change the rules.

Yet, there are some PCPs who seem to be accomplishing wonderful things for their patients and for themselves despite a reimbursement system that rewards procedures far more than thinking and wisdom, and that places a disproportionate set of administrative burdens on the clinicians who are least able to afford them. How is this magical outcome possible? In short, these clinicians have exploded the catch-22 in the only way one can do so: they have changed the rules. By this we mean they have stepped back and said, "Why should we keep doing things the way that we have always done them and expect a different (better) outcome?" (Albert Einstein has said that to persist in actions and expect a different outcome is the definition of insanity!) They have freed themselves from the hamster wheel by fundamentally changing how primary care is organized, delivered, and, in some cases, financed. We will devote a portion of this book to an exposition of the tasks of primary care in the context of relationship-centered care. We will demonstrate that the problems and harms we heard can be understood as failures of the tasks of primary care, and that these failures can in turn be understood as symptoms of basic design flaws in the processes for performing the tasks. As others have said, primary care in the US and other countries was for most of our history designed to respond to acute care needs, for there were no preventive measures and no effective tools for chronic disease management until relatively recently.[58] Yet the way most offices are designed reflects a model that is centuries old and not up to the tasks of modern primary care. We will present a variety of models of primary care that achieve what the Institute for Healthcare Improvement has called the "triple aim"—superior patient care experience, greater efficiency, and better population health.[59] We will present a synthesis based on these models that can allow the average US PCP to transform her practice from a place of low morale, chaos, and mediocre to poor performance to a triple aim model—what has come to be called a "patient-centered medical home," and do so without special outside financing.

Before we turn to our analyses and suggestions, we share, in Chapter 2, a representative sample of the stories we heard from the patients we interviewed. These narratives have been created from the interviews so as to portray a more coherent story, uninterrupted by interviewer questions. We have taken care, however, to maintain the fidelity of the narrative with the original interview, and hope that they can more fully communicate the preventable problems and harms these people experienced in their primary care. For the interested reader, we close this chapter with a representation of the introduction, methods, and results of the study that yielded these narratives.

INTRODUCTION

The report by the IOM *To Err is Human: building a safer health system*[1] focused public attention on the problem of medical error. It also stimulated policy-makers to devote new resources to characterize and prevent medical errors across the spectrum of health care. Much of the effort to date focuses on improving patient safety in hospitals, an appropriate priority given the suggested incidence of errors in inpatient settings,[60–62] the resulting anxiety engendered in the public sector,[63] and the opportunities for system redesign that can reduce the risk for errors and harms.[64] Yet most medical care occurs in ambulatory settings provided by primary care clinicians.[65,66]

Published information about medical error in ambulatory primary care settings is limited.[4,67–69] It focuses on errors in diagnosis, treatment, and the delivery of preventive services and suggests that a cascade of information transfer problems is the proximal cause for many of these failures.[70] Although important, these studies have serious limitations, including varied definitions of error, reliance upon physician reports and perspectives, inconsistent taxonomies of errors and harms, and an absence of the causal analyses advocated by human factors experts.[13]

Based on existing data, the prevailing perception is that medical errors endanger patients primarily through adverse drug events and surgical mishaps. Whether such errors pose the predominant threat to patients is unclear, however, because of the paucity of good epidemiological research. A fundamental source of uncertainty is whether the operational definitions of error used in patient safety studies and error surveillance systems are designed to capture the kinds of errors and harms that matter most to patients. The classic hospital-based studies of medical errors[60–62] dealt with injuries that prolonged the hospital stay and produced disability at the time of discharge. The scope of harm experienced by patients is clearly broader, however, and it almost certainly differs between inpatient and outpatient settings.

Relatively little work has been done to understand the patient's experience of medical errors in either setting. Large national and regional fixed-response surveys of the general population have been conducted.[7–10] Such surveys in the US have documented that medical errors and dissatisfaction with care are common experiences and that public perceptions about errors appear to differ from those of clinicians, but the surveys leave largely unanswered the specific nature of the errors and associated harms that consumers experience. Even less is known about the specific patient experience in primary care settings. This lack of knowledge hinders efforts to design, implement, and evaluate patient-centered care.

We report a qualitative study of primary care patients based on in-depth interviews to understand their experience of medical errors. Our specific aims were to develop patient-focused typologies of medical errors and associated injuries (or harms) in primary care settings; to understand from patients' perspectives which of these errors and injuries are most in need of correction; and to provide a basis for other research that will investigate error epidemiology, causes, and prevention. Additional aims, which we do not report on here in any detail, were to compare and contrast the patient's descriptions with reports of errors solicited from physicians and to construct simulations or guide observation of actual practice, with a goal of correcting system problems that predispose to the most important errors.

METHODS

Trained telephone recruiters used random-digit dialing to solicit adult respondents who received their care from general internists or family physicians, or whose children received their care from pediatricians or family physicians, in rural, urban, and suburban communities in Virginia and Ohio. Between 10 and 20 completed calls were required to recruit one respondent. Most solicitation calls were answered by female adults. To obtain our goal of one-third male respondents, we sometimes obtained support for the study from a female adult and asked her to solicit involvement from a male adult household member. Respondents were told they would contribute to a federally funded study of problems in primary health care. They were offered $50 to participate in the interviews, which lasted approximately 45 minutes and were conducted at the individual's home or another mutually convenient location. Three African-American women were trained as interviewers and were selected for their ability to relate well to persons from diverse socioeconomic groups. We reasoned that a male or white interviewer might inhibit the spoken communication of some respondents. The interviews were audiotaped and transcribed, and personally identifiable information was deleted.

The interviewers used an interview guide to solicit narratives of preventable incidents in primary care that resulted in a perceived harm. This framework was chosen to fit the following broad definition of error (favored by the investigators for this exploratory study): all forms of improper, delayed, or omitted care that unnecessarily injures patients by either worsening health outcomes or causing physical or emotional distress. Incidents that were not preventable, but were believed by our respondents to be inevitable consequences of care, were not coded as errors. Respondents were asked to describe both the incident and the harm with as many additional stories as they could recall. A cue card listing steps in primary care (telephoning the office, checking in for an appointment, being brought back to the examination room, etc.) prompted respondents to remember a range of incidents.

When all individual incidents were reported, the respondent was asked to group them according to which were the most and least disturbing. The interview also included questions regarding the duration of the relationship with the clinician and the demographic characteristics of the clinician and the respondent. Based on analysis of the initial interviews, subsequent respondents were asked to characterize their relationship with the clinician and probed for any perceived discrimination based upon race, age, sex, or ability to pay. The research protocol was reviewed and approved by the Office of Human Subjects Protection of Virginia Commonwealth University, and all respondents signed informed consent forms. A detailed exposition of the research proposal to the AHRQ, including the interview guide and cue card used for the study, has recently been published.[3]

The two principal investigators (AJK and SHW) independently performed the initial analysis of each interview, using an editing style of analysis.[71] In this method, one acknowledges previous constructs and assumptions but explicitly checks them against the data, making necessary modifications as the investigation proceeds. The analysis was concurrent with data acquisition[72] and created cumulative and prioritized lists of medical errors and harms. The investigators also looked for possible linkages between the themes of the stories and respondents' characteristics (e.g. sex, race, occupation) or clinician characteristics (e.g. specialty, sex, race).

A five-member consulting team with expertise in qualitative research design, medical psychology, medical sociology, critical theory, and error analysis provided ongoing critiques of the quality of the coding, the taxonomy construct, and the linkage to existing knowledge about patient experiences of medical error. Ecological validity (explicit and implicit norms and understanding shared by members of a community)[73] and authenticity (incorporating notions of fairness and a raised level of awareness)[74] were promoted by sharing the analysis with three reactor panels (focus groups) of 6 to 10 patients each, recruited from urban, suburban, and rural communities in the two states.

With input from reactor panels and consultants, and with an eye toward linkage with the developing literature on medical errors, we derived a taxonomy of patient-reported errors organized around five domains: access breakdown (desired care blocked or delayed), communication breakdown (failed transfer of information), relationship breakdown (deficiencies in patient-centered care), technical error (slips, lapses, or violations), and inefficiency (needless waste of resources). Although the interview guide was designed to make the harm associated with every incident explicit, it was not always possible to discern explicit harm from the narratives, and the investigators chose not to infer harms when not stated.

RESULTS

Forty-one individuals agreed to an interview, and 40 interviews were completed. Two interviews (African-American respondents from urban areas in Ohio) were unusable because of technical audiotape problems. Of the 38 usable interviews, 11 were from rural, 11 from suburban, and 3 from urban Virginia communities; the Ohio interviews occurred in seven urban and six suburban settings. Twenty-nine respondents were female, and 29 were African-American. The remaining respondents were white. Ages ranged from 21–77 years (median 38 years), and socioeconomic stratification (based on years of education, where stated) put 18 respondents in an upper class (more than 12 years' education), 13 in a middle class (9–12 years' education), and five in a lower class (fewer than nine years' education). The 38 narratives described 221 problematic incidents, most of which patients linked to specific harms. The incidents fell within 70 fourth-order categories (i.e. fourth layer of the taxonomy; 46 third-order categories are shown in Table 1.1), including errors of omission and commission, and occurred in all phases of primary care.

TABLE 1.1 Unique events associated with preventable harms*

			Instances of unique reports		
		Taxonomy order:	1st	2nd	3rd
1	Access breakdown		63		
	1.1	Difficulty initiating contact with office by telephone		10	
	1.2	Excessive delay in obtaining appointment with clinician		10	
	1.3	Excessive delay in obtaining referral to specialist		1	
	1.4	Excessive delay in / no return of phone call		7	
	1.5	Excessive office waiting time		17	
	1.6	Service not covered		11	
		1.6.1 Medications not covered			2
		1.6.2 Family member excluded from practice			1
		1.6.3 Specialty services limited			8
	1.7	Service not available		7	
		1.7.1 Lack of telephone care			4
		1.7.2 Lack of acute care			2
		1.7.3 Lack of evaluation before referral			1
2	Communication breakdown		17		
	2.1	Within office		8	
		2.1.1 Insurance information not recorded			1
		2.1.2 Insurance information not updated			1
		2.1.3 Payment not posted			1

(*continued*)

* To third order of taxonomy. Full taxonomy out to fourth order available from the authors upon request.

			Instances of unique reports		
		Taxonomy order:	1st	2nd	3rd
	2.1.4	Appointment improperly scheduled			3
	2.1.5	Wrong chart used for patient			2
2.2		Between office and outside entity other than patient		9	
	2.2.1	Referrals not done			4
	2.2.2	Improper coding of service			1
	2.2.3	Medication refill not called to pharmacy			2
	2.2.4	Records not transferred to requesting clinician			2
3		Relationship breakdown	82		
3.1		Inadequate time with clinician		9	
3.2		Intermediary imposed on communication with clinician		6	
3.3		Care by other than usual clinician		4	
3.4		Disrespect or insensitivity		63	
	3.4.1	Evident in interpersonal communication			38
	3.4.2	Evident in patient flow in office			20
	3.4.3	Evident in office environment			5
4		Technical error	54		
4.1		Deficiency in history		4	
	4.1.1	Incomplete history of present illness		2	
	4.1.2	Incomplete history of medications		1	
	4.1.3	Incomplete past history		1	
4.2		Deficiency in physical exam		1	
	4.2.1	Incomplete physical exam		1	
4.3		Deficiency in investigations		1	
	4.3.1	Artifact introduced in X-ray		1	
4.4		Deficiency in diagnosis		11	
	4.4.1	Failure to appreciate severity/acuity of problem		1	
	4.4.2	Wrong diagnosis		4	
	4.4.3	Dismissing selected symptoms		2	

(*continued*)

	Taxonomy order:		Instances of unique reports		
			1st	*2nd*	*3rd*
	4.4.3	Perceived failure to make any diagnosis			4
4.5		Deficiency in treatment and follow up		35	
	4.5.1	Poor injection technique			1
	4.5.2	Results of investigations not shared with patient			6
	4.5.3	Inadequate patient education re procedure, diagnosis or treatment			18
	4.5.4	Premature recommendation for hysterectomy			1
	4.5.5	Perceived polypharmacy			1
	4.5.6	Wrong medication dose			2
	4.5.7	No treatment for pain			2
	4.5.8	Inadequate follow-up care			4
4.6		Deficiency in business practice		2	
	4.6.1	Requiring patient to pay before insurance company			1
	4.6.2	Balance billing by participating clinician			1
5		Inefficiency of care	5		
	5.1	Excessive data elements for registration		1	
	5.2	Duplicative registration		2	
	5.3	Unnecessary office visit		2	
Total events			**221**		

Box 1.1 provides illustrative excerpts, organized in the order of the primary care experience, to portray some of the most common and most troubling problems. (A larger set of selected quotes is available in Appendix 1, which is online only as supplemental data at www.annfammed.org/cgi/content/full/2/4/333/DC1.)

BOX 1.1 Problems throughout the process of care

Trying to get through

So, I'm still getting the voicemail at 10:30 that says the office hours are 9–5. Please call back during work hours. [. . .] So I called again around 11:30, and I got a busy signal. Then the line was busy for like an hour straight 'cause I kept hitting repeat dialing. So, then I finally got through at 1:00 in the afternoon, and I was put on hold for like 45 minutes . . . And I didn't want to hang up because it had been such a difficult time getting through, so I'm just steady holding the phone.

African-American female, urban Ohio[1]*

Getting through to somebody, to a professional health care worker, was almost impossible . . . you get non–health care people answering phone calls, and I don't know if they are trying to screen them, I, I don't know, I don't know if they're busy . . . they never called me back that entire day, and I had to call, end up calling them back.

36-year-old white female pharmacist technician, suburban Virginia[2]

Checking in

You go to the window, you knock on the window and you stand there, and you wait and there's someone sitting at the window. You knock again, no answer. When you finally do get an answer from this person that's sitting there at the window, they've got attitude. They don't use a professional manner . . . talking down to you like you're a nobody. Like you're taking up their time. Like you're not a paying customer. Like you're disturbing them.

53-year-old African-American disabled male, urban Ohio[3]

They treat everybody like a new patient, and that is not necessary. It's like a waste of time because they ask too many questions, but if they pull my folder, they can see everything that I have just said, everything that they have just asked me about.

33-year-old African-American female business manager, suburban Ohio[4]

Waiting to be seen

I sat in the waiting room, and, ah, 45 minutes later I hadn't been called back . . ., so I went up and asked what the problem was, you know, did you forget I'm out here? And they said, no, no, we will be with you as soon as we can, the doctor's just busy today . . . so finally the nurse comes out and calls my name. I go back in the room, I get all undressed, get on a gown, and I'm sitting up here on the table, and an hour goes by, and a doctor hasn't come in yet. So, at that point, I get up, I put my clothes back on, and I walk out. When I first started going there, they had a little sign hanging up in the, in the waiting room that says, "If we have not called you in 15 minutes, please come to the desk," and, you know, question it. The sign's gone now.

White female medical receptionist, suburban Virginia[5]

I feel like, when you go in for an appointment, I don't feel that who I am should have anything to do with me being seen by a doctor, but I have seen people come in that are white, and they go right in to their doctor, and I've seen the lobby, be sittin' there, and there be a whole bunch of black people sitting there, and they just be sittin' there longer, and longer, and longer.

41-year-old African-American female clerical worker, rural Virginia[6]

The visit

When I go . . . when I go there . . . I mean it's this quick, boom boom boom. You know they've got so many people. They're running you in, they're running you out. And, you know, so, you've got to try to remember everything you need to say before your time is up.

39-year-old white female nurse, rural Virginia[7]

They need to talk to you about the medicines you are going to take, they need to know what other medications you are on. You know, they, sometimes they don't even ask, and they don't even look at your file.

32-year-old white female executive assistant, suburban Virginia[8]

The doctor really wasn't listening to what I was saying, and it was like, I kinda told him what happened and he already had his mind made up about what happened, and I was trying to tell him that I didn't think that was it. I mean, I'm not a doctor or anything, but you kinda know what's going with your body. . . . If he had just listened more to what I had to say [. . .].

24-year-old African-American male computer worker, urban Ohio[9]

Follow-up and referrals

I knew I had borderline cholesterol problems, and my father had just had quadruple bypass, and I thought, you know, I had better get this checked out. I went in, they never called me about my results. My cholesterol was 300, and 200 is the, kind of the, you know, don't go past this mark. They never called me, they never followed up with any sort of recommendation.

36-year-old white female pharmacy technician, suburban Virginia[10]

I said I want to see a specialist, and I said I would feel much more comfortable if I go to a specialist myself just to see me to see what the problems are, and he reluctantly done it but acted like it's a, he told me I really didn't, you know, need to, and I don't think he should never tell me what I need to do.

64-year-old African-American male corrections officer, urban Ohio[11]

*Typology codes:

1 Access breakdown, difficulty contacting office, involving telephone system, telephone not answered, and excessive time on hold.
2 Relationship breakdown, intermediary imposed on communication with clinician; and access breakdown, no return of telephone call.
3 Relationship breakdown, disrespect or insensitivity, evident in interpersonal communication, rude behavior.
4 Inefficiency of care, duplicative registration.
5 Access breakdown, excessive office waiting time.
6 Relationship breakdown, disrespect or insensitivity, evident in patient flow in the office, prioritizing patients based on race.
7 Relationship breakdown, inadequate time with provider.
8 Technical error, deficiency in history, incomplete history of medications.
9 Relationship breakdown, disrespect or insensitivity, evident in interpersonal communication, patient advice ignored.
10 Technical error, deficiency in treatment or follow-up, results of investigations not shared with patient.
11 Relationship breakdown, disrespect or insensitivity, evident in interpersonal communication, patient preferences not respected.

The most common incidents involved breakdowns in the clinician–patient relationship (n = 82, 37%) and in access to clinicians (n = 63, 29%). Patients' descriptions of breakdowns in the clinician–patient relationship were dominated by stories of disrespect or insensitivity, which accounted for 63 (77%) of the 82 incidents. Three kinds of problems accounted for 58% of the reported breakdowns in access (n = 63): difficulty in contacting the office (n = 10, 16%), delays in obtaining appointments (n = 10, 16%), and excessive office waiting times (n = 17, 27%). Technical errors such as misdiagnosis or adverse drug events were reported less frequently (n = 54, 24%) than were relationship and access breakdowns. The incidents involved 170 reported harms, which fell into 40 categories (Table 1.2). Fully 119 (70%) of the 170 harms were psychological. Within this category patients were most likely to report anger (n = 31, 26%), frustration (n = 17, 14%), belittlement (n = 15, 13%), and loss of relationship with and trust in their clinician (n = 18, 15%). Pain and avoidable personal expense were the most commonly mentioned physical and economic harms, respectively. When asked toward the end of the interview to rank the incidents in terms of importance, most respondents emphasized technical failures of misdiagnosis, failure to disclose test results, and inadequate patient education; relationship breakdowns involving rude staff, disregard for patient concerns, and racial bias; and access breakdowns created by long waits for appointments.

TABLE 1.2 Preventable harms (n = 170) reported by respondents, by number of unique instances

Harm	Instances
Psychological	119
Anger and related emotions	
Anger	31
Upset	8
Irritated	4
Frustrated	17
Personal worth	
Belittled	15
Sense of violation	3
Sense of betrayal	1
Relationship effects	
Diminished trust in clinician	11
Diminished relationship with clinician	7
Anxiety about health	10
Related to opportunity cost	
Wasted time	6
Anxiety about other responsibilities	2
Anxiety about bills	2
Forget important issue	1
Other emotions	
Disappointed	1
Confused	1
Mood swing	1

(*continued*)

Harm	Instances
Physical	39
Pain	
Not otherwise specified	12
Abdominal pain	2
Low back pain	1
Bruising	4
Related to medication effects	
Hypoglycemia	2
Somnolence	1
Drug interactions	1
Worsening problem	
Asthma	3
Hypertension	1
Cellulitis	1
Flank abscess	1
Uterine bleeding	1
Undertreated, untreated conditions	
Hyperlipidemia	1
Diabetes	1
Sjögren's syndrome	
Other	
Weakness	2
"Sick"	2
Dizziness	1
Fever	1
Economic, other	
Avoidable personal medical expense	9
Threat to credit rating	1
Lost work time, pay	1
End of sports career	1

The sample size and the qualitative coding of the data do not lend themselves to a statistical analysis of associations. Careful readings of the narratives, however, did not reveal any apparent patterns with respect to the sex or specialty of the clinician, duration of relationship, community type, state, form of health insurance, or the age, sex, and imputed socioeconomic status of the patient. The only obvious association with any characteristic was with respect to stories of apparent racism, which were heard only from African-American respondents and which were found in stories from rural, suburban, and urban communities in both Virginia and Ohio.

Our reactor panels—the groups of people with whom we shared interview excerpts linked to our tentative coding scheme—validated our labels for the errors and told us that both physical morbidity and serious psychological harms were very important. They also noted that seemingly trivial insults could eventually lead to more serious problems and that even near misses could cause anxiety and diminished trust. Several members suggested that some of the errors might be due to offices being too busy, to physicians that are inadequately trained or who have not maintained their competence, to prejudice, and to the unintended consequences of managed care.

REFERENCES

1 Kohn LT, Corrigan J, Donaldson MS. *To Err is Human: building a safer health system.* Washington, DC: National Academy Press; 2000.

2 Kuzel AJ, Woolf SH, Gilchrist VJ, Engel JD, LaVeist TA, Vincent C, *et al.* Patient reports of preventable problems and harms in primary health care. *Ann Fam Med.* 2004 Jul–Aug; **2**(4): 333–40.

3 Kuzel AJ, Woolf SH, Engel JD, Gilchrist VJ, Frankel RM, LaVeist TA, *et al.* Making the case for a qualitative study of medical errors in primary care. *Qual Health Res.* 2003 Jul; **13**(6): 743–80.

4 Dovey SM, Meyers DS, Phillips RL, Green LA, Fryer GE, Galliher JM, *et al.* A preliminary taxonomy of medical errors in family practice. *Qual Saf Health Care.* 2002 Sep; **11**(3): 233–8.

5 Makeham MA, Dovey SM, County M, Kidd MR. An international taxonomy for errors in general practice: a pilot study. *Med J Aust.* 2002 Jul; **177**(2): 68–72.

6 Layde PM, Maas LA, Teret SP, Brasel KJ, Kuhn EM, Mercy JA, *et al.* Patient safety efforts should focus on medical injuries. *JAMA.* 2002 Apr; **287**(15): 1993–7.

7 National Patient Safety Foundation at the AMA. *Public Opinion of Patient Safety Research Findings;* 1997 September. Available at: www.npsf.org/download/1997survey.pdf (accessed January 16, 2010).

8 Henry J Kaiser Family Foundation. *National Survey on Americans as Health Care Consumers: an update on quality information;* 2000. Available at: www.kff.org/kaiserpolls/3093-index.cfm (accessed March 23, 2003).

9 Robinson AR, Hohmann KB, Rifkin JI, Topp D, Gilroy CM, Pickard JA, *et al.* Physician and public opinions on quality of health care and the problem of medical errors. *Arch Intern Med.* 2002 Oct; **162**(19): 2186–90.

10 Blendon RJ, DesRoches CM, Brodie M, Benson JM, Rosen AB, Schneider E, *et al*. Patient safety: views of practicing physicians and the public on medical errors. *N Engl J Med.* 2002 Dec; **347**(24): 1933–40.

11 Committee on Quality of Health Care in America, Institute of Medicine. *Crossing the Quality Chasm: a new health system for the 21st century.* Washington, DC: National Academy Press; 2001.

12 Lee TH. A broader concept of medical errors. *N Engl J Med.* 2002 Dec; **347**(24): 1965–7.

13 Vincent C, Taylor-Adams S, Chapman EJ, Hewett D, Prior S, Strange P, *et al*. How to investigate and analyse clinical incidents: clinical risk unit and association of litigation and risk management protocol. *Br Med J.* 2000 Mar; **320**(7237): 777–81.

14 Vincent C. Understanding and responding to adverse events. *N Engl J Med.* 2003 Mar; **348**(11): 1051–6.

15 Institute for Healthcare Improvement. *Conferences and Seminars*; 2010. Available at: www.ihi.org/IHI/Programs/ConferencesAndSeminars (accessed January 16, 2010).

16 Murray M, Tantau C. Same-day appointments: exploding the access paradigm. *Fam Pract Manag.* 2000 Sep; **7**(8): 45–50.

17 Adams WG, Mann AM, Bauchner H. Use of an electronic medical record improves the quality of urban pediatric primary care. *Pediatrics.* 2003 Mar; **111**(3): 626–32.

18 Safran DG. Defining the future of primary care: what can we learn from patients? *Ann Intern Med.* 2003 Feb; **138**(3): 248–55.

19 Murphy J, Chang H, Montgomery JE, Rogers WH, Safran DG. The quality of physician-patient relationships: patients' experiences 1996–1999. *J Fam Pract.* 2001 Feb; **50**(2): 123–9.

20 Swick HM, Szenas P, Danoff D, Whitcomb ME. Teaching professionalism in undergraduate medical education. *JAMA.* 1999 Sep; **282**(9): 830–2.

21 Accreditation Council for Graduate Medical Education. *VI. Resident Duty Hours in the Learning and Working Environment*, from http://acgme-2010standards.org/pdf/Common_Program_Requirements_07012011.pdf (accessed January 18, 2010).

22 Elder NC, Vonder Meulen M, Cassedy A. The identification of medical errors by family physicians during outpatient visits. *Ann Fam Med.* 2004 Mar–Apr; **2**(2): 125–9.

23 Phillips RL Jr, Bartholomew LA, Dovey SM, Fryer GE Jr, Miyoshi TJ, Green LA. Learning from malpractice claims about negligent, adverse events in primary care in the United States. *Qual Saf Health Care.* 2004 Apr; **13**(2): 121–6.

24 Woolf SH, Kuzel AJ, Dovey SM, Phillips RL Jr. A string of mistakes: the importance of cascade analysis in describing, counting, and preventing medical errors. *Ann Fam Med.* 2004 Jul–Aug; **2**(4): 317–26.

25 Rosser W, Dovey S, Bordman R, White D, Crighton E, Drummond N. Medical errors in primary care: results of an international study of family practice. *Can Fam Physician.* 2005 Mar; **51**: 386–7.

26 Bird S. Missing test results and failure to diagnose. *Aust Fam Physician.* 2004 May; **33**(5): 360–1.

27 Poon EG, Gandhi TK, Sequist TD, Murff HJ, Karson AS, Bates DW. "I wish I had seen this test result earlier!": dissatisfaction with test result management systems in primary care. *Arch Intern Med.* 2004 Nov; **164**(20): 2223–8.

28 Hickner J, Graham DG, Elder NC, Brandt E, Emsermann CB, Dovey S, *et al.* Testing process errors and their harms and consequences reported from family medicine practices: a study of the American Academy of Family Physicians National Research Network. *Qual Saf Health Care.* 2008 Jun; **17**(3): 194–200.

29 Casalino LP, Dunham D, Chin MH, Bielang R, Kistner EO, Karrison TG, *et al.* Frequency of failure to inform patients of clinically significant outpatient test results. *Arch Intern Med.* 2009 Jun; **169**(12): 1123–9.

30 Elder NC, McEwen TR, Flach JM, Gallimore JJ. Management of test results in family medicine offices. *Ann Fam Med.* 2009 Jul–Aug; **7**(4): 343–51.

31 Gandhi TK, Weingart SN, Seger AC, Borus J, Burdick E, Poon EG, *et al.* Outpatient prescribing errors and the impact of computerized prescribing. *J Gen Intern Med.* 2005 Sep; **20**(9): 837–41.

32 Kuo GM, Phillips RL, Graham D, Hickner JM. Medication errors reported by US family physicians and their office staff. *Qual Saf Health Care.* 2008 Aug; **17**(4): 286–90.

33 Smith PC, Araya-Guerra R, Bublitz C, Parnes B, Dickinson LM, Van Vorst R, *et al.* Missing clinical information during primary care visits. *JAMA.* 2005 Feb; **293**(5): 565–71.

34 Elder NC, Hickner J. Missing clinical information: the system is down. *JAMA.* 2005 Feb; **293**(5): 617–19.

35 Kripalani S, LeFevre F, Phillips CO, Williams MV, Basaviah P, Baker DW. Deficits in communication and information transfer between hospital-based and primary care physicians: implications for patient safety and continuity of care. *JAMA.* 2007 Feb; **297**(8): 831–41.

36 Singh R, Servoss T, Kalsman M, Fox C, Singh G. Estimating impacts on safety caused by the introduction of electronic medical records in primary care. *Inform Prim Care.* 2004; **12**(4): 235–42.

37 Elder NC, Pallerla H, Regan S. What do family physicians consider an error? A comparison of definitions and physician perception. *BMC Fam Pract.* 2006 Dec; **7**: 73.

38 Makeham MA, Kidd MR, Saltman DC, Mira M, Bridges-Webb C, Cooper C, *et al.* The threats to Australian patient safety (TAPS) study: incidence of reported errors in general practice. *Med J Aust.* 2006 Jul; **185**(2): 95–8.

39 Solberg LI, Asche SE, Averbeck BM, Hayek AM, Schmitt KG, Lindquist TC, *et al.* Can patient safety be measured by surveys of patient experiences? *Jt Comm J Qual Patient Saf.* 2008 May; **34**(5): 266–74.

40 Kostopoulou O, Delaney BC, Munro CW. Diagnostic difficulty and error in primary care: a systematic review. *Fam Pract.* 2008 Dec; **25**(6): 400–13.

41 Dowell D, Manwell LB, Maguire A, An PG, Paluch L, Felix K, *et al.* Urban outpatient views on quality and safety in primary care. *Healthc Q.* 2005; **8**(2): S2–8.

42 Van Vorst RF, Araya-Guerra R, Felzien M, Fernald D, Elder N, Duclos C, *et al.* Rural

community members' perceptions of harm from medical mistakes: a High Plains Research Network (HPRN) Study. *J Am Board Fam Med.* 2007 Mar–Apr; **20**(2): 135–43.

43 Wetzels R, Wolters R, van Weel C, Wensing M. Mix of methods is needed to identify adverse events in general practice: a prospective observational study. *BMC Fam Pract.* 2008 Jun; **9**: 35.

44 Wasson JH, MacKenzie TA, Hall M. Patients use an internet technology to report when things go wrong. *Qual Saf Health Care.* 2007 Jun; **16**(3): 213–15.

45 Taylor BB, Marcantonio ER, Pagovich O, Carbo A, Bergmann M, Davis RB, *et al.* Do medical inpatients who report poor service quality experience more adverse events and medical errors? *Med Care.* 2008 Feb; **46**(2): 224–8.

46 Bagian JP. Patient safety: what is really at issue? *Front Health Serv Manage.* 2005; **22**(1): 3–16.

47 Halpern J. *From Detached Concern to Empathy: humanizing medical practice.* New York: Oxford University Press; 2001.

48 Stone JH. What are we all but patients? *Reconstructing Empathy: the heart of relationship-centered caring.* Akron, OH: Institute for Professionalism Inquiry; Nov 18, 2005. Available at www.summahealth.org/media/10157/14511.pdf

49 Engel JD, Zarconi J, Pethtel LL, Missimi SA. *Narrative in Health Care: healing patients, practitioners, profession, and community.* Oxford and New York: Radcliffe Publishing; 2008.

50 Suchman AL, Markakis K, Beckman HB, Frankel R. A model of empathic communication in the medical interview. *JAMA.* 1997 Feb; **277**(8): 678–82.

51 Roter DL, Hall JA, Merisca R, Nordstrom B, Cretin D, Svarstad B. Effectiveness of interventions to improve patient compliance: a meta-analysis. *Med Care.* 1998 Aug; **36**(8): 1138–61.

52 Kim SS, Kaplowitz S, Johnston MV. The effects of physician empathy on patient satisfaction and compliance. *Eval Health Prof.* 2004 Sep; **27**(3): 237–51.

53 Stewart M, Brown JB, Donner A, McWhinney IR, Oates J, Weston WW, *et al.* The impact of patient-centered care on outcomes. *J Fam Pract.* 2000 Sep; **49**(9): 796–804.

54 Roter DL, Stewart M, Putnam SM, Lipkin M Jr, Stiles W, Inui TS. Communication patterns of primary care physicians. *JAMA.* 1997 Jan; **277**(4): 350–6.

55 Stewart M, Brown J, Weston W. Patient-centred interviewing part III: five provocative questions. *Can Fam Physician.* 1989 Jan; **35**: 159–61.

56 Beach MC, Sugarman J, Johnson RL, Arbelaez JJ, Duggan PS, Cooper LA. Do patients treated with dignity report higher satisfaction, adherence, and receipt of preventive care? *Ann Fam Med.* 2005 Jul–Aug; **3**(4): 331–8.

57 Morrison I, Smith R. Hamster health care. *BMJ.* 2000 Dec; **321**(7276): 1541–2.

58 Fox DM. *Power and Illness: the failure of American health policy.* Berkeley, CA: University of California Press; 1993.

59 Berwick DM, Nolan TW, Whittington J. The triple aim: care, health, and cost. *Health Aff (Millwood).* 2008 May–Jun; **27**(3): 759–69.

60 Brennan TA, Leape LL, Laird NM, Hebert L, Localio AR, Lawthers AG, *et al.* Incidence of adverse events and negligence in hospitalized patients: results of the Harvard Medical Practice Study I. *N Engl J Med.* 1991 Feb; **324**(6): 370–6.

61 Wilson RM, Runciman WB, Gibberd RW, Harrison BT, Newby L, Hamilton JD. The quality in Australian health care study. *Med J Aust.* 1995 Nov; **163**(9): 458–71.

62 Thomas EJ, Studdert DM, Burstin HR, Orav EJ, Zeena T, Williams EJ, *et al.* Incidence and types of adverse events and negligent care in Utah and Colorado. *Med Care.* 2000 Mar; **38**(3): 261–71.

63 Agency for Healthcare Research and Quality. *Survey Shows that Medical Errors and Malpractice are Among Public's Top Measures of Health Care Quality.* Press Release. Rockville, MD: Agency for Healthcare Research and Quality; December 11, 2000. Available at: www.ahcpr.gov/news/press/pr2000/kffsurvpr.htm (accessed January 16, 2010).

64 Reason JT. *Human Error.* Cambridge and New York: Cambridge University Press; 1990.

65 White KL, Williams TF, Greenberg BG. The ecology of medical care. *N Engl J Med.* 1961 Nov; **265**: 885–92.

66 Green LA, Fryer GE, Yawn BP, Lanier D, Dovey SM. The ecology of medical care revisited. *N Engl Med.* 2001 Jun; **344**(26): 2021–5.

67 Ely JW, Levinson W, Elder NC, Mainous AG, Vinson DC. Perceived causes of family physicians errors. *J Fam Pract.* 1995 Apr; **40**(4): 337–44.

68 Fischer G, Fetters MD, Munro AP, Goldman EB. Adverse events in primary care identified from a risk-management database. *J Fam Pract.* 1997 Jul; **45**(1): 40–6.

69 Bhasale AL, Miller GC, Reid SE, Britt HC. Analysing potential harm in Australian general practice: an incident-monitoring study. *Med J Aust.* 1998 Jul; **169**(2): 73–6.

70 Robert Graham Center for Policy Studies in Primary Care. Toxic cascades: a comprehensive way to think about medical errors. *Am Fam Physician.* 2001 Mar; **63**(5): 847.

71 Miller WL, Crabtree BF. Clinical research: a multimethod typology and qualitative roadmap. In: Crabtree BF, Miller WL, editors. *Doing Qualitative Research.* 2nd ed. Thousand Oaks, CA: Sage; 1999. pp. 3–30.

72 Miller WL, Crabtree BF. The dance of interpretation. In: Crabtree BF, Miller WL, editors. *Doing Qualitative Research.* 2nd ed. Thousand Oaks, CA: Sage; 1999. pp. 127–43.

73 Cicourel AV. *Method and Measurement in Sociology.* New York: Free Press of Glencoe; 1964.

74 Guba EG, Lincoln YS. *Fourth Generation Evaluation.* Newbury Park, CA: Sage; 1989.

CHAPTER 2

Seven stories

I WANT THINGS BACK TO THE WAY THEY WERE

I am a 42-year-old African-American woman who lives and works in Ohio. I hold down two jobs to make a living. I am both a corrections officer and a beautician. Among other illness I have diabetes and high blood pressure. I'd like to tell you about some of experiences I've had with my health care. Let me begin by sharing some background concerning my relationship with my physician, a female general internist.

When I didn't have insurance, my provider made a program with me where I paid so much a month until I did get a job where I did get insurance. That's one of the reasons why I stuck with her because she was very caring. At first I wasn't a good patient. I didn't take all the medicine that she gave me, because I am not a medicine taker. I would prefer to go another route than to take the medicine and that might have made her frustrated, but I am not one that wants to take 8–10 pills a day. So I tried to find another alternative, but I would tell her if something affected me that I didn't like and that I discontinued the use and asked to try something else. Maybe that disappointed her or maybe made her upset where she didn't want to just give me the care because she knew I wasn't going to do it anyway. So you know I just want her to care about me. You know, she's pretty good; it's just a few things that need to change. She always was very lenient and she would talk with me, but it just seems apparent right now that she might be overloaded or she just might be tired right now. She needs to rest because she is not giving me the care that she had been giving me over the years. And, it is making me a little bit upset and frustrated because she did give me top A care and now it seems like she is getting a little lax on it, so it's making me very upset. I want things to be back the way they were. So now, let me describe experiences with my internist and her office that have troubled me and brought me to this point. I'll begin with some experiences with office staff.

The "killer secretary" as I call her was very nasty when she first started. She was very nasty and she didn't listen to things that you were saying when you were at the doctor's office. She was so rude and nasty at the time I couldn't get an appointment or anything else because she was so nasty. I don't know what she said to the doctor, but the doctor asked me to be much nicer and to have patience with her. But, it was really the secretary who didn't have patience with her customers. She showed a lack of compassion for those she dealt with and her treatment made me very upset. I talked to the doctor about this and she must have talked with the secretary because she developed a better attitude.

Getting an appointment is really difficult and frustrating. Just recently I did call about getting an appointment, and the secretary did not ask me whether it was urgent or not, and she gave me a much later appointment than I really wanted. I needed one much earlier than that and I had to call her back and tell her that because she didn't even ask. I am still waiting for an appointment. I would call it the appointment from heck, because I am still sick and I need to be cared for right away. I think this harmful act is due to the lack of the nurse even trying to find out what my problem was. If it was serious or it was something I could have waited for. She just didn't even try to find out. I think it needs to be fixed because someone might have something very, very serious and if they don't try to find out, then it might be too late. You know, they might die waiting for the appointment. And so, they should try to find out everything they possibly can before they consider what appointment you are going to have, try to find out what your health problem is and then they will know how to schedule your appointment. Problems like this can be fixed. She should have tried to talk with the doctor and see if she could speed up my appointment and get me in earlier to make sure that everything would be all right, especially with diabetes and plus I was on a new medication. I think she should have called me, she should have called back or just told me that she would call me back, asked me some questions and then conferred with the doctor and then called me and made the appointment. She could have even left it on the answering service to let me know if it was all right because I might have needed to get in right away. The significance of this experience is very important to me.

Referrals have been another problem. When the doctor wants me to go to a specialist and they say they are going to call me for an appointment with the specialist and I never get the call, or when I go back I have to remind them of a lot of things the doctor gave me. I have to remind them of things to do that they forgot and they will tell me, "Let's wait till next time." But, it will still never get done. This is very frustrating to me. So much so that right now I have been considering going to another doctor because I feel like the doctor really is not having my best interest at heart and it's making me feel like I am paying my money for nothing. And I really want to get the best care that I can. I feel that if I called the doctor's attention, as well as her staff attention to some of the errors that they have made, maybe they will correct them and make it better for future references or times for appointments. Make it better for other people that may call in so that they are being cared for properly. If they would make a change and show me that they are trying to change, you know to get it right, because other than that again it makes me want to just move on to someone else.

One thing I will say is that the office staff are pretty good on phone calls. You know they don't put you on hold a whole lot or anything like that, they usually take your call right away or if you leave something um, on the answering service they do get back to you.

Let me tell you a little about my troubling experiences with the doctor. Once I got inside the doctor's office room and they forgot me. They were getting ready to close-up and go to lunch. I had to call out to them and remind them that I was in the doctor's office. So they had to call the doctor back because she was getting ready to leave and remind her that they had forgotten about me. I don't know if it was being in a rush or an oversight, a mistake, or they were rushing her in to get some lunch. But, I had been in there for hours. I really just can't understand how she passed my room and went to everybody else and left me. It really made me highly upset. But because I felt that she was a good doctor, I decided to give her another chance. I think this error was probably due to the nurses neglect to inform the doctor that I was there or even remind her. This was very significant to me. But to be fair, I should tell you that they did come right in and they called the doctor back and the doctor came and she checked me and everything, and they did apologize and they were very kind about it and asked for my forgiveness.

One time the doctor was talking to another one of her patients in another exam room. She was really loud with the patient and she was talking about her business and I thought the doctor should have been more cordial or quiet because I heard all of her medical business. I thought the doctor could have been a little bit more professional in the way she talked and watched that other people didn't listen in on the conversation. I wonder what causes something like this. Maybe the doctor was tired or she was frustrated with her patient because she wasn't following her directions to a T. But, she knows she should have been a lot more discrete with her patient so that other people wouldn't hear their business. Whatever the problem was, her and that patient needed to solve it and not everybody else in the building—doctors lack discreteness sometimes. This type of thing troubles me. I was hoping that nobody would hear my business when she come in. I was worrying. I said that I was hoping that I would be last so that wouldn't nobody hear my business 'cause she was pretty loud. She has a private office which she might have used. If she wanted to talk to the lady she could have took her into her office and closed the door so that the other patients wouldn't hear what she was saying to the lady.

You know, appointments can be very disappointing and this is very harmful. Every time after I get into the room usually the nurse asks me what my problem is and she writes it down before the doctor comes in. Well, after the doctor comes in and you know how you try and at least write a list down or put on your remembrance a lot of things that have been going wrong since the last time you have seen her. Well, when you see the doctor the first she tells you is one thing at a time and you never get to tell the doctor the rest of the things. She just treats one thing and throws others off until later. Other things might be very important to you, but she doesn't want to treat more than one to two things. She just stays in a hurry and just knocks it off or disregards what you are saying and just tells you give me one to two things and that's it. What causes this? Sometimes the doctor, I think is tired and maybe she needs a vacation because it is like she just can't handle all the stress and she just wants you to make her day lighter by telling her just a little bit of your problem and not all of it. Such treatment made me very upset because I felt like that I was going to doctor for no reason, to no avail. It wasn't accomplishing anything because when I went there I couldn't tell her all of my problems and how I was feeling. So, I don't feel like I was being diagnosed right because, I didn't give her everything that I had to put together so she could diagnose me properly. I tried to talk to the doctor, but she just flagged me off. She was like just give her this and that and then she was off on her way. If she would have listened to everything that I said and then treated me as such and not just got part of it then she wouldn't have treated just what she thought was the problem.

Another time I remember a machine was cut off by accident. It needed to stay on throughout the day so it would be ready for my appointment. I guess it took time for it to warm up. I don't know if it was a sonogram, I think it might have been a sonogram or something like that or the EKG. The doctor came in and she was fussing at the nurse and the nurse was very upset and she was trying to tell the doctor that she didn't turn the machine off, but the doctor didn't want to listen to her or anything she had to say. She just went in on the girl and was fussing at her in front of me and everything and the nurse was very upset and I was too. I really didn't appreciate the way she treated her. She was trying to tell her she wasn't the one who turned it off and she didn't know how it happened, but the doctor wouldn't listen to her, she just kept running her mouth and fussing and it made me upset even with the doctor because she didn't listen to the nurse and I thought that wasn't professional either. I thought she was really harsh with the young lady. It made me very upset and I felt sorry for the staff. It would have been easy to handle this situation in a more professional manner by taking the nurse in the office or pulling her aside and talking with her and getting a true understanding. She just didn't. She just assumed.

Sometimes physicians prescribe too many medications. For example, she gives me a lot of different medicines. I don't like to take all those different medicines. Not too long ago I told her about some medicine that she tried out on me for my diabetes and a lot of my hair came out. So, she in turn said that I don't need to get so many hair relaxers. She knows that I am a beautician, but she thinks I get too many relaxers which cause my hair to break off. She is saying the cause is too many perms in my hair. Too many perms, instead of trying to find out if that was it. Then she changed me to another medication which I am taking now and I had to stop taking. Well I went to her and I told her that the medicine was making me excessively eat. Now I was keeping my diabetes down, but now I just eat, eat, eat, and I started gaining weight. I told her that I was gaining weight. The medicine does say that you should expect to gain 8–10 pounds once you start taking it, but I had exceeded 8–10 pounds and was going for more. My clothes were getting tight and I told her and she told me it was just the clothes that I had on. I also made an appointment to let her know that this medicine was making me swell and I was very jittery and I have to wake up all night long because my sugar count would drop real, real low. Well, I have not gotten in to see the doctor yet. So, I have just stopped taking the medicine and I think it has steroids in it so I did wean myself off of it. I think this error was due to the doctor's lack of interest or something. It makes me very upset and it could be helped by her monitoring me more closely with the medicine. She should have come in at least once a week or something or as much as my care provider would let me so that she could make sure that, especially this is a new pill on the market to make sure that it was effective and doing what it supposed to do.

I had also been having problems with my ear. I have been having a lot of ear aches and I swell up around the side of my face and all down in my jaw and my neck. She looked in it and she said it wasn't nothing but water build-up and it would be okay. But she never gave me a treatment or any medicine for it, and I am still having problems with it now. I have sharp stabbing pain, my balance is off, I have been having a lot of problems and she said it wasn't nothing serious. I really don't know why she doesn't understand. Maybe she doesn't think it is serious enough. She said it was from the sinuses or something, but I have been having very bad headaches and I have stabbing ear pain and sometimes it even causes me not to be able to work because it hurts so bad. I think this could have been helped by checking me over. My neck's been swollen, my shoulders, everything. I have trouble with my hands. I also told her about the burning in my hands and trouble with my arms and stuff because I am a beautician. She said I have carpal tunnel and that is it. You know what, I did go and get it checked years ago and I haven't had it checked any more. She did give me braces years ago and she is doing nothing about it, and it is progressing worse now. I think this is neglect and that's why I'm looking for another doctor. It's apparent that she doesn't care anymore. She should have sent me to a specialist or something to see what I could have done.

I hope that by telling my story it will make a difference with a lot of doctors, and make them more caring and attentive after the things that they do and do not do, so maybe it will make their practice much better.

WORRIED TILL THIS DAY

My name is Phyllis and I'm a single mom living in the suburbs of a southern city and working as a legal assistant. I have two children, Margaret and Max. I'd like to tell you a few stories about what it's like for me when I take the children to see the pediatrician. There are several pediatricians in the office and I've been going to the same place for about five years now. I pretty much see any doctor when I take one of the kids in, I'm not real specific on which ones they see. There is only one in particular who is kind of an up-front type of doctor so you don't get along with her all the time.

Sometimes I try to take care of things over the phone. Like when my son whose teacher had asked me to get his hearing checked. When I called the doctor's office I told them what I needed, they transferred me to this other lady who had to set me up with a specialist. It took her a week to call me back, and I ended up calling her back and leaving another message. The delay really caused a problem for me. Max's teacher actually got pretty upset with me and had some words with me because it took a while to get this done. Even after they referred me and everything, I still had problems as far as getting it paid for from the insurance company.

Getting test results is another problem. Margaret has a lot of urinary tract infections and needs lots of tests. I really can't stand their testing because what they do is they take what they need, and they send it across the street to get test results and then you don't get them. They'll tell you "okay, if you don't hear from us within five days or you can call us back." I mean, it just kind of leaves you in the wind, you know, I don't think that is very professional. I think they should, you know, give you a call to let you know. Like I said, Margaret has had to take a lot of tests for her tract infection to make sure it's not some kind of infection in her kidney. So the first time I called back because I wanted to know the results.

But you know, when it got to be a few times that she was going back for tests, I kind of waited to see if they were going to call me back. So when they don't that means nothing is wrong. But, during the period I'm waiting, I get frustrated and Margaret knows I get frustrated and I don't mean for her to know, but it's frustrating because I feel like I need an explanation so I can prevent it and it won't happen again, but, I mean, any time you take them in there, it's either a virus let it go, or, I mean, it's just, it drives me nuts. It's just hard watching your kid be in pain and then the doctors, I mean, I know they can't do everything as quick as snapping your fingers. I think the thing to do about these problems is get more help.

Another thing that is really frustrating when you go to the office is registration at the front desk. It never fails, you go in there, they ask who you are, they verify your address, verify your insurance information which has never changed every time you go in there. I kid you not. I've had the same insurance. I know I have updated this every time I have went in there, but for some reason and they always tell me, "Oh well we're updating our records," or "something has happened to our computers." You know it is always an excuse, but the insurance information never changes! The funny thing is, the person that does it, she has been there you know for quite a while. I know she can't remember everybody, but I just, I just don't understand, maybe it something to do with their computers, I don't know. I think they need a better computer system, maybe.

Now let me tell you about seeing the pediatrician. I haven't really had a problem with her except understanding the diagnosis. Margaret had a problem with her urine since she was about a year or two old. She had an extremely big amount of blood in her urine. I mean, it was really dark and the doctor waived it off as if she was having a menstrual cycle at a year or two old, at least that's the way I took it. Then one day I was at work and my mother-in-law at the time, she actually my best friend, called me because she was babysitting Margaret while I was at work. She witnessed what was going on because Margaret used the bathroom and there it was. It was just pure darkness. So, I rushed and I took her to the emergency room and let's just say they never gave me an answer to what was going on. To them, it seemed like it was no big deal. It cleared up. She never was given any medicine for it. Like I say, the doctor diagnosed it like it was no big deal. She made it seem like that they knew her body was flushing out like during a menstrual cycle. I just don't know. I guess I could have questioned her a little more, but I just took it as "Okay, you're the doctor," because I was a young mother and I took it as okay you know what you are talking about and that was that. Till this day, even when she has tract infections, till this day, I worry you know, because I don't know if something is like inside of her that's going to explode one day and all of this is because of that one incident from a long time ago, that still worries me to this day. Every once in a while she complains of stomach aches or stomach pain and that just worries me that there is something going on that they didn't detect when she was younger—all this blood in her urine. There's not really an answer in the diagnosis. I really haven't had a moment's peace. I'm, scared till this day, worried till this day. Yeah, I have a problem with their diagnosis. I just don't feel like they give you enough answers. I think they need to do a little more testing. I mean, I leave and then take her to the emergency room. From the pediatrician to the emergency room, they just both make it seem like no big deal. I just think a little more testing and a little more explanation of what is going on. But, as I told you, I figured, "Okay, you know what you are talking about." Now, however, as an older and wiser mom, I realize that if you question enough you'll get what you are looking for and I have gotten to the point where like in Margaret's situations, the reason I don't call back is because finally I got a doctor to explain to me that when the urine comes out red that's blood cells. So it kind of makes sense to me why there is blood in the urine. I think once you sit down and totally understand the explanation that helps. I think a person like me who doesn't understand medical terminology or exactly what you're saying, a doctor who is talking to a parent who doesn't know the right questions to ask, could just be more specific, something more close to the truth.

Another thing I'd like to tell you about is giving shots to kids. I understand doing them quick, but I think a lot of parents don't like the really harsh stab of it. You know, it's one thing to give it to them quick, but another thing to just pound it. When Margaret got her last shot, she lost it. I guess the quickness was good, but at the same time it was just too much for her. My son, he is terrified, he doesn't like it. You should at least let them know it's going to be OK and not jab so hard.

Don't you just hate insurance? I do! Personally I would like to say that as far as insurance is concerned, I think they should just all open up a savings account and let us put our money in there and then if we need it they can pay for it because it's our money instead of telling us that they can pay for it, or that they can't pay for it. I had this really awful insurance when I was married to my husband and they didn't want to pay for anything, nothing. And then you know, you go there, you sit there and you don't want to go through all this crap just to get them to pay this one bill, so it's kind of like forget it, I'm just going to pay it and be done with it. You know, it's often errors in the doctor's office that are made. The insurance company would tell me, "Well you doctor's office didn't bill this right, they didn't put the right code," or something like that. You would talk to the doctor's office. The doctor's office would tell you, "Well we billed them this, and oh you're right, we didn't put the right code," or then it will still come back not paid, so you call them back. "Well the insurance company still didn't put the right code," and that's when you just go, "Okay, forget it." I give up, you know, because I feel like they want to sit there and argue with you and argue with you and until you say forget it. This makes me feel uncomfortable when I go into the doctor's office knowing that I owe them money and I don't feel like I should be paying, I mean, I pay my co-pay you know, and that is what I expect to pay.

One of the things I'd find really helpful is a follow-up call after a visit because then that way you don't have to call the doctor's office to report this is still happening. You know that way the doctor or nurse can call you and if you have any concerns you can tell them. But, if everything is fine, it's a quick phone call, "Everything is fine. Thank you for calling." That would be nice, you know, because that way you don't have to sit there and leave messages for the doctor or nurse to call you. I used to work for a pharmacy, and if anybody would come in with a prescription for an antibiotic, we would call that person back in two weeks because normally antibiotics are good for 10 days. You would call that person back. We had a list that would print out every two weeks. We would call them to see how they were doing and they could talk to the pharmacist if they had any questions or concerns. I think if the doctor or nurse would call that would be awesome because they would know more.

ATTENTIVE CONCERN AND RESPECT FOR PATIENT

As a 64-year-old African-American male I have a number of stories I want to share with you. I'm a diabetic with high blood pressure. My wife and I see the same general practitioner and have for several years. I work in the State corrections system and have good health coverage. I'd like to tell you about our experiences with our doctor and his office.

Our doctor's office is always crowded and so you have to wait for a long time to get an appointment and then when you go there you have a long wait even with an appointment, usually an hour or two. Our doctor is okay and I have a fair relationship with him. But, his staff, especially the receptionist, has an attitude that irritates me. She seems like she can't be bothered helping you. I remember one time my wife was ill and she was throwing up. She had started throwing up at like 1:00 in the morning, so during the morning at about 9:00 she told me that she hadn't yet stopped. I called the doctor's office and I said I have to get her in because she is really throwing up. The receptionist was very nasty to me on the phone. She said, "We can get her in today after 2:30. I said, "But, I mean, she is really ill." "We still can't get her in until 2:30," she said. I said, "Well I'll just take her to the emergency room," and she said, "Well take her then," and that really irritated me mostly because of the fact that she has been going there for so many, many years and then all of a sudden, you have a new receptionist that just blows you off. This really took away a lot of the professionalism they had before. Even if she couldn't get us in I think it could have been handled a lot better than just to tell me go to the emergency room. I mean, it's like you're nothing. You know, the biggest thing that day was just to get her to the doctor and get her the medicine. For me it also hurt because I mean, you put trust in your provider, and then that happened. There was no reason for this treatment because a lot of times you can tell people things that they might not want to hear, but you could tell them in a very professional manner, which they could understand. She could have very well said, "You know, we are very booked, we're packed. Why don't you take her to emergency." I think they forgot about that, you know. In that field you've got to have a human side and it's just not pills and shots. I mean, there is a human side which I think she forgot about—she forgot about the good part of it. Because of this treatment I was thinking for a little while of switching doctors.

Another thing that disappoints me is how the office handles prescriptions. If I run out I have to go into the office. I think they are just after the $15 co-pay. It makes me go a different route to get my medication. So, I mean, instead of going to the doctor and get a prescription, I just go through my company, and get it three months at a time, that way I don't have to worry about it. So I find a way around it rather than call the office. As I've thought about this, I think sometimes the doctors are so wrapped up in how many patients they can see that many things get put on the back burner. As far as the patient calling and asking for something, it's just that, you know they get their 15 minutes with you, 10 minutes with you and that's it. Meanwhile, it seems like they cram so many people in that they don't have time for you. They could have just called it in to my pharmacy. They could have very easily took 5 or 10 minutes and called up my pharmacy and, then I just go pick it up.

One of my greatest disappointments as I look back on my care was I told the doctor, "I'm so thirsty all the time," and I guess it didn't register with him. I kept telling him how thirsty I was and how much I was going to the bathroom. He took too long to diagnose what was wrong with me. Then I had a blood test and he says, "You are borderline diabetic." Afterwards, I found out there is no such thing, it's either you are or you aren't. For that year and a half that I was going through it, my legs were killing me, my back was killing me. I couldn't even walk up and down the steps. Like one step at a time. That's how bad I was hurting.

My quality of life at that time was bad. Everybody thought I was spoiled. Well, I mean, you don't feel like doing anything and I think a year and a half of that could have been avoided.

Once he decided, found out I mean, that I was actually a diabetic I went on the medication and exercised and stuff and now it's like better, 90% of it went away. Another thing that bothers me is that at first he didn't explain the consequences of the disease or the side-effects of the medication. He didn't tell me about diet or exercise. Being a doctor you should know about diabetes especially in an African-American minority. It angered me. I would expect my doctor to know more about me as a patient and my culture, and how bad diabetes is for me as a black male. I wonder how to explain this late diagnosis. I don't know if it was neglect or lack of knowledge. I got more information off the internet than I got from him. Sometimes I think it would be better seeing specialists. But, I do think that he could have taken a little more time and really looked at me and listened to what I was telling him. Sometimes you wonder if you go and talk to them that they just go through the motions and they write it down and just go on about their business, you know to the next patient. I think that they got to listen to what the patient is saying. I think if he would have done more listening to what I was telling him that he could have diagnosed my diabetes a lot sooner. After all is said and done, I think I would have got a little more confidence if he would have just said, "You know, I think it took a little long." If he'd have just come out and said that he missed the signs I would have gotten a little more confidence. I think that would have helped me because even right now I still think about all that time that I spent hurting. And, I am mad, very mad, I mean, it just makes you angry.

Getting referrals is another issue I have with my doctor. One time I told him I was having a little pain and I want to go see a urologist and he tells me, "Well you don't really need to go see a urologist." I said, "But I want to go see a urologist. I would feel much more comfortable if I go to a specialist myself just to see what the problems are." He reluctantly done it but acted like it's unnecessary. I don't think he should ever tell me what I need to do. I think if I request to go see a specialist, then his job is to give me a referral. It makes you wonder if he, if doctors, are really hiding stuff from you. I mean do they get worried that they did miss a diagnosis.

I need to tell you about how, in my experience, minorities are treated when they go to a hospital. This is important because a lot of our community are minorities and they get their health care from the hospital emergency room. Every time a black person or minority walks in, they assume that we don't have health care, and that assumption just bothers me to no end. You know, I have a very decent job. I have a very good health care coverage and it just irritates me that when I walk in they assume that I don't have it or else that my wife don't have it. You can't assume that every black person that walks into an emergency room is on welfare—that's stereotyping. You can't take one minority and use them to judge all minority people just like you can't use one white person to judge all white people. This takes away my dignity and I don't want anybody to do that. Where I live, as a minority you are constantly dealing with white doctors, white providers and I don't think they know how to interact with you. This goes for doctors' offices too. I think they have to be more educated in how to deal with minorities. When 90%–95% of a doctor's patients are white and 5% may be black, he doesn't really understand about black peoples' views sometimes. It's just a lack of knowledge and that should change.

PREJUDICE, CONFUSION, AND LITTLE TIME
I want to tell you my stories about health care because I think they can matter for us all. I'm Marsha, a 26-year-old African-American living in the Midwest and working at an agency that provides youth services. I've been seeing the same PCPs for about eight years now. Our relationship is mixed—sometimes good and then sometimes not so good. She cares for my low blood pressure, chronic asthma, my thyroid, and irregular menstrual periods.

So let me begin with my experiences with her office staff. There's been a change in staff and the one lady and I had problems. She had a very nasty attitude. She wouldn't allow me to speak with the doctor because at the time my bill was overdue and I was sick and off of work and had trouble paying it. She was upset because I wasn't paying the bill the way she wanted me to so she didn't allow me to speak to the doctor. And when I called to the doctor to let her know I was bringing in a whole payment instead of the lady listening to me she made me come in. I think the lady was very arrogant. She didn't have time to listen. She basically felt like that we weren't paying so she wasn't going to get paid and instead of her finding out what the problem was and trying to see how to correct it, she brushed you off. At the time when I called her, I had the money to pay her and a couple other family members' bills that I wanted to pay. But instead, she was very ignorant instead of listening. So that made me have to take time off of work and have to come in. It caused a lot of confusion. I was upset by this. It hurt my feelings that the lady treated me the way she did because, you know, I still showed her respect, the utmost respect even though she treated me the way she did. She had to be spoken to about her behavior and it even cut in on the doctor's time of taking care of other patients because she had to come in and correct the situation that could have been dealt with offhand. This was so upsetting to me that for a moment I did go see another physician because I was upset about her staff, but I had to realize it wasn't her fault. She always had been good to me so I came back to her.

I remember one time I messed up my right foot, my right ankle and my mother went with me to the doctor's office. They didn't want to take care of us right away and the odd thing is that they kept taking white people instead of the black people in the office. Maybe five or six people came in after us and they wasn't serious as me and this other black person, but they were taken. The office person could have come in and spoke to us and gave us some reason so there would be closure to the situation. Even if they were telling a story they could have made it look like they weren't being prejudiced. So, I waited so long that I had to go to the bathroom. Well, I'm in the bathroom and the sink fell onto my left foot so then I get emergency attention real fast. I think it was because they were worried about a lawsuit. So they took me back and they didn't make us wait a long time. After they treated me my mother had to push me out in a wheelchair and it was icy outside. So it's really bad, and we were sliding down the street in this wheelchair and the ice was all around. It seems funny today but back then it was really bad. It made me angry because I'm the type of person that treats everybody equally. I don't care what you look like. Waiting all that time in the office, if a person went before it should have been a priority because they were more serious and should get faster care. But that wasn't the case and it made me upset.

Probably the most serious problem I had with my physician was when she mixed me up with my aunt. Me and her look very similar. So when she came talking to me about different things in my file, she was talking to me about my aunt's information. And I'm not my aunt, so I was confused. Then she said, "Oh," and left and didn't even say she'd be back. She just left and I didn't see her for about a half an hour to an hour. I mean, we have problems because she was mixing up me and my aunt's file. I knew her information and she probably knew my information, you know. I felt that she didn't take proper care, like she was too busy and had too much on her mind. My aunt and I resemble each other but I don't think we look that much alike. The doctor was giving me personal details. She came in talking to me about my ovaries and they weren't even my ovaries she was talking about. Not mine! And I was looking at her like she was crazy. I said, "I got what!" I was confused and I was worried. I think that sometimes doctors take on more than they can handle and they need to sometimes take a vacation and realize what's going on with theirselves. Well, when she came back, she just started talking to me about my stuff. She could have apologized or explained to me what was going on. But she seemed in her own world. And at one point I looked across the room to the exam room on the other side of the hallway and saw my aunt and we waved to each other! I suppose what upsets me the most about this is that somebody else's personal business was told to the wrong person. They may not want anyone to know and being that I knew the person and we were family members, that was embarrassing 'cause maybe she didn't feel that she wanted anybody to know that she had that problem and at that time she felt, you know, her confidentiality was breached.

Oh, let me tell you about the problem with my prescription. My doctor had blood work done 'cause she was looking for diabetes. So they did all my blood work and I had them fax all my files to her so when I went to see her everything would be there. So, she looked over my blood work and then she drew more blood and had me come in for another appointment. She said, "Well for a big girl you have excellent blood work. I can't understand why you're so healthy." I said, "I can't, either." So she said, "Well then I'm going to put you on Glucophage." She said, "You are not a diabetic, understand this." She said, "This will help you with your irregular menstrual and with your weight." But, what I was trying to find out basically if I had thyroid problems because I have all the symptoms. Well she gave me this medicine. My sugar already stayed between a 100 and 120, and she knows my blood pressure stays low sometimes. She gave me about 1000 mg a day and I was feeling like I was passing out and so she said, "Just break the pill in half," instead of coming in, instead of checking my blood to find out why I'm dropping so low. She told me I was producing too much estrogen and that makes me produce too much sugar. I said, "I don't know what you're talking about. You have to break these down for me. I don't know what's going on." She just loved to experiment with medications and different things. She had me on steroids, prednisone and then said to me she don't know why I gained weight and she gave me medicine on top of medicine and I was just, just confused. I was upset because the medicine had me going through mood swings that affect me as far as working with my job. I work with the public, I work with children and it's hard to control yourself when you're on medication because one minute you're up and the next minute you're down and then it's like you got kids that you work with and they have different attitudes and personalities so you're clicking out on them trying to control the medicine at the same time and you got to maintain your total self with working. It just wasn't working. I was upset and being that she was my doctor, I felt that she was right so I listened to her. Then I came to my senses and realized that they're not always right even though they're a doctor and I started to wean myself off the medications so I wouldn't harm myself. Because eventually, I felt that maybe I'd have a bad effect from it. You know, through it all, I think that she thought she did as much as she could to assist me. But, I felt that she didn't do as much as she could have done because she didn't take the time. Once again it's time with her. She didn't take the time to find out what my problem was and sit down and go over my charts and everything because I was there giving her everything. I was going to different doctors having to fax everything over to help her out but it's like she really never had the time and it's like now that she has more patients she don't have the time she had when she had a little bit of patients. No time and too many patients. It's hard for her to see so many of us who are scheduled at the same time. Come to find out that most of us wait for an hour or two after we get there for our appointment. For me it's really hard. I do a 12 hours shift so I would have to cancel the time from my work. I'm on a point system so we didn't have any sick days or doctor days and I lost points on my attendance and also got my pay docked. Another thing I was there for half a day so a half of my days was gone even if I had any other important things to take care of. Actually, it has gotten worse. That's a lot of reasons why I haven't went back to her. She's an excellent doctor but now that she has more patients, it's hard, it's hard to get the quality care that she had given me when I first went to her.

I think it's good to tell these stories. It's a good thing because a lot of people don't find out that these are really problems that occur. And, they don't take them serious. They think it's just something that's common and occurs every day. And, you know, nobody takes things like this serious. They like, "Oh well they happen and you will get over it." But, this is something that really happens and is a serious problem. People do have legitimate concerns and questions about it and if people would take the time to listen they would find out that a lot of these simple problems actually escalate to bigger things and it could be that they could be solved at a lower level before it gets so big.

WHERE IS THE COMPASSION?

Ted is my name and I'm a 53-year-old African-American and I no longer work because I'm out on permanent disability. I've been going to the same general practitioner for about 20 years. Getting in to see one of the two doctors is really hard. The phone lines are always busy. Once you do get someone, you could be put on hold for an unlimited, unspecified time. It's hard to get a hold of the doctor most of the time. You can't speak directly with the doctor. They say the doctor will call you back. It may be the next day sometimes before you hear from him. When you call you have a problem and you can't get anyone to handle it at that time. It definitely upsets me. And, it seems to me that if they would staff the facilities with people to handle situations all this could well be avoided. But you know, talking to my friends, getting an appointment seems to be a problem at most physicians' offices. You need an appointment right away. You may not get it for a week. The senior citizen I help take care of was having a problem with breathing. She was having shortness of breath and I needed to speak with the physician to find out exactly what to do. I spoke with the nurse. She said that she would call me back within the half hour. She didn't. I waited something like maybe 90 minutes and ended up taking my senior to the emergency room. It makes you really angry, very perturbed not knowing what to do next. I feel that this is the result of too many people handling too many jobs. If the office was staffed with personnel to handle problems that come up on the spur of the moment then that problem wouldn't exist.

I suffer with chronic back pain. I remember one time that I called to get an appointment. I had seen the doctor once. I had medical advice and medications but I was having a real problem with my back. I was at the point I couldn't barely move. I needed to see a doctor right away and I couldn't get in. I was told that the doctor was filled up and that I would have to possibly go to emergency. Going there would entail for me seeing someone that didn't know my history, didn't know my problem, didn't know my meds. I'd be there for hours on hours and, again, I feel that could have been avoided. Emotionally and physically I was already a wreck. It didn't help that I wasn't getting any help. There's no compassion in this way of treating people. I felt betrayal on their part. My being a patient, not a new patient but a patient, an established patient, I should have been treated a little better than I was. Well anyway, I ended up going to emergency and staying. I think I was there about five hours with only directions to follow-up with my physician. And again, I waited days for an appointment. So, I was suffering in the meantime. As I've thought about this, it seems to me that I could have possibly been made the last patient of the day. Someone could have talked to the doctor who may have prescribed a stronger med for me knowing my problem. I probably could have been prescribed a stronger medication, something to at least relieve the pain until such time as I could have been seen. And once you do get in, you just wait. One time I was having real problems with sitting down. I couldn't sit very long and then to sit in the office, well, I was hurting more when I got to see the doctor than when I came in. I asked the receptionist, "How long will it be before the doctor came in." I told her, "I've been sitting here quite awhile and I'm really starting to hurt," and her reply is something I won't forget, "Either you wait or you leave." It's like she's doing you a favor letting you sit in the doctor's office.

It seems like no matter what doctor you go to see there are problems. I take my grandchildren to see their doctor. At the front registration desk, they have a closed window. It's not clear glass and so you can't see through it. You go to the window, you knock on the window and you stand there and you wait and there's someone sitting on the other side of the window. You knock again, no answer. When you finally do get an answer from this person that's sitting there at the window, they've got attitude. They don't use a professional manner. They talk down to you like you're a nobody; like you're taking up their time; like you're not a paying customer; like you're disturbing them. It's just unprofessional and it makes my frustration boil. All you want to do is sign the registration sheet and it's on the other side of the window where you can't get to it! And once you do finally get to sign in, you just sit and wait. This other time I took my grand-children in for an 8:30 appointment, signed in and then sat there with an office full of people for two and a half hours before the doctor came in. Then it was, wait for the doctor. Finally they call you in, the nurse gets blood pressure, that's what she has to do, and she sits you in the exam room and you wait still. You spend on average four, four and a half hours seeing the doctor. It makes you very angry. It makes a lot of people very angry. You've got people sitting and waiting with scheduled appointments and a doctor not there and a staff that won't try to explain to you what's holding him up or where he is. Well, eventually I changed my grandchildren's doctor.

Another thing about the doctor I see and I think many doctors is that they don't listen. Asking doctors questions and doctors not hearing what you're saying but telling you what they want you to hear happens all the time. Once I went in to have some tests done, an EMG, myelogram, and an MRI. I was just speaking with the doctor after all of these procedures were done and he was explaining to me what they had come up with out of everything they'd done. I proceeded to ask him questions about one particular thing about one of the X-rays that he was showing me and his reply was, "I just told you what that was." I let it go. I asked another question as to the myelogram and his reply was, "This is what I just told you," but it wasn't what I had asked him. Here again he wasn't listening to what I was asking him. He was telling me what he wanted me to know, but he wasn't answering my questions. He wasn't telling me what I wanted to know. I think the error with the physician is that he feels that his prognosis is good enough for his patient; whether the patient has a question or not. He feels that what he says should have been understood fully without someone asking. Or it could have been that he felt holier-than-thou, "What I've told you should be sufficient and that's that." I was so frustrated. And all it would have taken to help me was to just explain things to me and answer any questions I had for him.

I guess all my experiences with the doctors and the staff in their offices has convinced me that all doctors and staff need much more training in how to deal with other people.

RUNAROUND AND FRAGMENTATION: FRUSTRATED WITH THE WHOLE SYSTEM

Sue's my name and I'm 32 years old. I have a great job as the executive assistant to the president of a restaurant chain. My family and I go to an HMO for our health care. Mainly I see the doctors for headaches and high blood pressure. For the last 18 months I've been dealing with high blood pressure issues with a specialist and two of the doctors in the HMO, but more about that later. Access and treatment in this system add a lot of frustration and tension to my life.

Getting referrals are the one thing they do really well. If you call for a referral, you're voice prompted through the voicemail to this one lady who's very efficient, and she handles all of the referrals. That's the one good thing about this office. But voicemail to get an appointment is a whole other story. You know, it's irritating. Most of the time, by the time I call my doctor I've been sick all night and waited to 8:30 to call, and you can't get through until like 10:00, and at that point you don't really want to talk to a machine. You have waited long enough, you want to talk to a person. I mean, it's just so irritating to have to go through voice trees, if you want to get a prescription refilled, if you want to get a referral, if you want to make an appointment. And the first thing they say is, "If it's an emergency dial 911." I probably would have thought of that in an emergency! And when you get through and you want to make an appointment they normally cannot see you. The one thing that bothers me the most is they do not tell you that you are not seeing your physician. You might see any of the six doctors that are in there, and you don't know until you get there that that's who you are seeing. So the whole time your thinking that you're going to see your doctor, the one who knows me, and then you get in there and you're seeing someone new that has never seen you before, and doesn't know your history, hasn't read your file. He just knows you're coming in for a blood pressure check and has no clue what medication you're on, or that you need to change your medication, or anything like that. That is really irritating and dangerous. And then, when you get there, you have to wait an hour to see a doctor. So, you're waiting an hour to see a doctor that isn't your doctor. They really can't help you when you get in there because he doesn't know your situation. And this is a normal occurrence. When I try to request my physician, I'm told he's too busy. He's either too busy taking walk-ins, or they have double-booked his appointments. The walk-ins are taken regardless of when they come, whether there's an appointment or not. The walk-ins are worked in between appointments. So you might wait an hour for your appointment because the doctor's taken three walk-ins, even though you are there early, I'm always there like 15 minutes early and I never get to see the doctor in under an hour. I start asking at 20 minutes, "Am

I next?" And if it's 20 minutes, and they're getting ready to take me, she'll say, "Well they're doing really great today. They are only behind an hour." That's just so irritating, because I've had my appointment on the books for three months. And then when I get there, it's not with my doctor! You know, you would have thought that if I see my doctor and he tells me come back in a month, and I go straight to the receptionist desk and make an appointment, that she'd make it with him and not just any doctor in the office. It's very frustrating. It just makes you wanna change, but finding a new doctor is so difficult, especially with an HMO like I have. So, I don't want to change doctors' offices too much, but when someone asks you who your primary care doctor is, I give them the name of my insurance card, because I don't know who it is anymore, I see whatever doctor sees me. It's really irritating, it bothers me a lot. I would say it's a major concern with the health industry today. And what's more important, it absolutely affects my blood pressure. I'm so frustrated by the time I get in there because it's taken so long and I need to get to work. I've got a cell phone and beeper going off. People need me. My time is just as valuable as theirs. I've got a life to get back to, that's why I made an appointment. It's always up when I get in there. I monitor it every day at work and it'll be, you know, somewhat high. By the time I get in that doctor's office it is sky-high. One doctor was afraid I was gonna have a stroke, and made me lay down until it came down. He gave me two medications to get it down, this is crazy. I guess they are doing the best they can. I just need to not get so upset. I try not to put myself in situations where I'm helpless, but the situation in the doctor's office makes me feel almost violated. They are in control and there's nothing you can do, not even for your own medical care. But the good news is that they have a new doctor there and she is wonderful. I requested a specific doctor before and have been told, "No, you can't see him," but now I will wait to see her. It'll make my day worse but at least I know that I have to wait and at least I know who I'm seeing when I wait.

The front office staff doesn't help matters. There's nothing helpful about them. There is a crotchety old receptionist that you have to go through. You know, the first impression you get is your impression of the whole office. I get a bad impression every time I go in there because she is the first thing you see, and the first thing you have to deal with, and there is nothing helpful about her, nothing. Like this time when I had been waiting for over 40 minutes and this elderly man, he was probably in his 70s, had been there even longer. He went up to ask if he was next, and the receptionist said, "Well no, you're not next, but if you're here for a flu shot we don't have any." I was sitting by the receptionist's desk, and I heard this. He asked, "Well do you know where I can go to get one?" She said, "NO." So I looked at the elderly gentleman, who obviously needed his flu shot, and I said, "Sir, I think I heard that Patient First has shots, so let me call." I looked at her and said, "Do you have a phone book?", and she said, "There is one on my table out there." So I looked up Patient First and I said, "Do you have a phone?" "Well there's one over there," she tells me. So I called Patient First, and they had shots. I told the man where it was located, and he thanked me, he was very appreciative. The man was never angry or anything, he was just upset that the receptionist treated him that way. So I sent him on his way, and she looked at me, and she had the nerve to ask me, "Where was that for the shots?" I just said, "You should have picked up the phone at 8:00 this morning when you knew you didn't have any flu vaccine, and helped these people to find some other place. These are patients; these aren't people off the street that are here to bother you." She doesn't see the importance about a receptionist being in customer service; she's in a hospitality position.

Another minor thing, but it's important, is the state of the doctors' office. The first thing you notice is how chaotic it is. Everybody's ticked off that they've waited so long, except for the walk-in people who are just so sick. Maybe they need to clear one doctor's schedule to see walk-ins, and not schedule him appointments. But, everybody is so irritated; it is so chaotic around there. The phone rings and rings before they answer it. And, they have an aquarium that makes a whole lot of noise that it is not supposed to. So, between that noise, the phone ringing, people disgusted because they sit out there for so long, it's just chaotic. And, that is very frustrating in that office. Most of the time people are sick and I think that you need to provide a nice environment for them. A simple "Ma'am, it looks like it's going to be about 20 more minutes until he sees you." Or, "The doctor has had an emergency." Just let people know that they are not sitting there in perpetuity for the rest of their lives.

Let me tell you what happened when I took my husband for his first full-blown physical. The doctor comes in and says, "Okay, we are gonna do a physical," and then the nurse comes through and she runs you up and down the hall, either height-ing or weight-ing you, or getting you to pee in a cup. You really don't know what they are going to do next, which is very uncomfortable. I mean, you literally feel like cattle being put through the maze of the slaughter because you don't know what's at the end of the thing. My husband had no idea that they were going to bend him over, and he didn't know that was coming, even when they bent him over he thought it was just like a cough test or something, and they surprised him, so he felt a little violated when we walked out of there. You shouldn't have to tell them to explain to you what is going on. So, that was probably one of the worst experiences for him. He's not one that wants to jump up and go to the doctor anyway. That was pretty bad. It's a frightening thing to be in the doctor's office or a hospital and not know what is going to happen to you. Somebody just needs to turn around and talk to you.

Speaking about talking to the patient, let me tell you another thing that's so difficult in dealing with my doctors. When you go to your doctor, they might tell you that you have a virus. He doesn't know the name of the virus, and that's fine, but don't just glaze over it. I'm the kind of person that likes to know what's wrong with me. I like a diagnosis, and, unfortunately, I have one of those doctors that says, "Okay, you're sick." But, I like to know what's wrong with me. I understand that they can't always do that, but at least you need to make a person feel validated, that they're more than just sick, you know, that it's a real thing that's wrong with them. They do need to explain it to you. They need to talk to you about the medicines you are going to take. They need to know what other medications you are on. Sometimes they don't even ask, and they don't even look at your file. I've had to have my pharmacist tell me that my doctor is giving me drugs related to my high blood pressure that you should not take together. I said, "Well my doctor says to take them," and she said, "Okay, well then we'll give them to you." I don't think the doctors are reading the information in my chart. It was two doctors in that office that put me on these two prescriptions, and it was in the same file. It's because I see a different doctor every time. They don't know, they don't read to see what I'm already on. I didn't know to tell them that I was on the one drug. I thought they knew since it was right there in my file. So, I'd switch doctors a whole lot quicker than I'd switch pharmacists, because she is probably keeping me alive. I called the office to tell the doctors about this. I left a message that I was on the two drugs, and the nurse called me back and said she thought that would probably be okay. So that's why I'm still taking them today. Now, as far as doctors communicating the information about my blood pressure problem I had one of my doctors that I saw in that office tell me to get off birth control. Well I have other problems where I can't be off of that because of severe heavy bleeding. So, he said to call my gynecologist and tell him you can't take it. I called my gynecologist and he said, "Well I don't know what else to do, maybe, you're on the strongest pill that they make, maybe we need to do a hysterectomy." So I called back to my doctor to tell him that, because they won't call each other. Then it just so happens that I go in the office and have to see a different doctor the next time, and she says, "Well no, we don't need to take you off your birth control, we need to give you a blood pressure pill." The other doctor told me I won't give you a blood pressure pill because you'll have a stroke as long as you're on the birth control. This is the kind of mess that goes on. The doctors won't pick up the phone and call each other, and get down to what's going on. They make me be the go-between, and

I don't know medicine. They'll say call your gynecologist and he told me that if your doctor says you can't take blood pressure medicine I can't give it to you. So, I call him back, well the other doctor says that you can. Who does he talk to when he calls? Does he call the doctor that doesn't want me to take it, or does he call the doctor that will let me take it? So I don't know who to let speak for my own care. I mean, obviously, I want to stay on the pill because I don't want to have the bleeding that I have, and I don't want to have a hysterectomy. So I'm going back about every month for them to tell me that my blood pressure is still high, and we need to do another pill. And the time that I left the doctor's office after he told me that I might have a stroke, I was physically sick and depressed. I told my husband, "I have a two-year-old baby and here I am, the doctor told me I could drop dead today." And when I go to the other doctor she says, Well you know it's high, but it's not that high." So there I was for a month I thought I was gonna die, and I came off my birth control, and bled for the next 15 days. I went back to another doctor and said we've got to do something. But still it's not resolved.

Well I want to end by telling you about the care for my child. My two-year-old is suffering through asthma, or allergies, or something. They are trying to diagnose what's wrong. I understand my doctor says that at that age it is hard to tell the difference between allergies and asthma, but if it's allergies she is awfully progressed for her age. I have been taking her for this problem since she was about eight months old. She has been going through these coughing spells and upper respiratory problems, and she will cough until she vomits. So I take her back, he puts her on the antibiotics for 10 days, she is better for 10 days, and then we are back in the doctor's office, back on antibiotics. So I finally was at my wits end a couple of months ago when I went in to the doctor, and I look at the doctor with tears in my eyes and said, "This is ridiculous. Either you're going to tell me what's wrong with her, and tell me that you cannot cure it, but will treat it, or either your gonna look at me and your gonna tell me that your gonna fix it, because I, I can't tolerate any runaround anymore." I said, "She's two years old and vomiting every day, and coughing every day, and it's become a way of life for her, and she accepts it." I said, "I will not tell her that this is the way her life is going to be until you tell me, but you have got to tell me something. We need to pee or get off the pot, and we need a diagnosis." So, he looks at me at the end of it, and I feel like I've been a little rude to him, but I don't mean to be, and says, "Well Sue, I really thank you for your frankness, and I want to let you know we will continue working on this until we get it down to a diagnosis. The first thing we are going to do is treat her for asthma." Well it just so happens that she got sick again last week and we took her back. Now they are treating her for the allergies. But I understand that you have to go through certain tests before they find out, but it amazed me that I had to be all but rude to the man for him to treat me like a human and look at me and do something. I hate that I had to go that far, and I hate that she had to be sick for 18 months before he took it seriously. Being involved in every part of the system is frustrating and brings more problems in addition to the one's you're trying to get help for.

INSURANCE-CONTROLLED CARE

My name is Joseph and I am a 54-year-old African-American. I work as shipping and receiving clerk, 12 hours a day, and seven days a week. I want to tell you about how I have to get my health care. There are two doctors, both internists, in the office but I see only one of 'em. I've been going there for 10 years for the simple reason that it's because of my job. We have certain doctors we have to go to see because of what the insurance company demands. If you keep your own private doctor they would not pay the bill. I don't like it because you are forced to go see a doctor that you don't particularly want to go to see. I look at it this way, it's my opinion, I'm not talking about everybody else. When you go to these doctors, they only do what they can do. Now my doctor told me, "I'm gonna treat ya, but I don't like the insurance carrier. Regardless whether I like it or not, I'm gonna still give you the same treatment as I would anybody else." But I notice if I go get a physical, or anything of that nature, it's the same physical as I get when I go to the company nurse for one, unless I ask for this or ask for that. The insurance tells 'em what he can and can't do. Another doctor was my physician before the company changed insurance and this man used to give me a great physical, the difference is just night and day. But I had to stop going to him because of the insurance. Now to get good treatment I have to ask certain questions. I go in there, the nurse comes in, she weighs me, she checks my blood pressure, and so on. Then you hear a knock and he comes in, he do the same thing, and he says, "Well, everything's all right." And I say, "Well, how was my blood? How was my sugar that last time I was in here? Or blood?" "Oh, yeah, that's right," he says, "Go get blood work before you leave today." I shouldn't have to be askin' all these things. He will not come right out and say, "Well last time you was here we did lab work, or whatever. No, I have to sit there and ask him if there was anything wrong. He should tell me how my blood sugar and high blood pressure are doin'. He should tell me that everything is fine or things are not checkin' out. It makes me angry with the way the rules and regulations are and you don't have much of a choice. My biggest problem was my blood pressure was up. I didn't need no doctor to tell me, I knew. The smoking will elevate your blood pressure. Drinking alcohol will elevate your blood pressure. Worry, a whole lot of things, stress, a lot of things, you know, will elevate your blood pressure. We don't talk about those things. But he does do pretty good with the medications.

You know, one time I had the flu and I went to see the company nurse. She said, "You need to get to the doctor," and told me to call my doctor. I told her I'd never get in. So she called and they told her I couldn't get in that day and she, being a registered nurse, I guess they listened to her and I got in. If it wasn't for her I would have waited a week.

I remember once they sent me to get X-rays. The doctor says, "Well, they have X-rays here in the facility downstairs." Well I had to end up paying that whole cost because my insurance company did not. These people were not part of the network and so they wouldn't pay. I think that if the office staff had more knowledge they should have let me know that I wouldn't be covered by my insurance.

I feel pretty much forced to go to the doctor that I go to and he is pretty much forced to see me. I don't feel we have a personal relationship and I don't feel that I get good care like I did before when I went to see the doctor I liked. It's frustrating for us all.

For those who may wish to use a live performance of the themes of these stories as an educational tool, please *see* Appendix 1.

CHAPTER 3

The heart of medicine

As foreground to the remaining chapters, we first set a broad and critical context for the work of reforming primary care practice. We believe that at its core, the practice of medicine is a relational and moral practice that is conditioned by the nature of illness and the responsive character of medical acts in the service of healing. In the current socio-political discussions of health care reform, it is easy to forget this philosophical and valued-based position. This is especially true in the face of passionate portrayals of scientific/technological advancements and new financial models for medicine as business, commerce, and corporation. This nexus—science-technology-finance—is advanced as the dominant strategy for improving the care of patients, the relationship between patients and physicians, and the relationships among health care professionals. To be sure, applications of current science, technology, and financial models are important considerations. However, in their overwhelming power as a change strategy, their resulting dominance easily transmutes the moral intent and force of ideas that place the patient center stage in reform debates, current ideas such as *patient vulnerability*, *relationship and patient-centered care*, *narrative health care*, and *the medical home*.[1-6]

Regardless of the particular form of social organization for medical practice, the patient–physician interaction has always been, and will always be, the core of the profession. Here we take our lead from the work of the eminent physician and philosopher, Edmund Pellegrino, who argues that three interrelated phenomena set the boundaries for medical activity: the nature of illness, the act of profession, and the end of medicine.[2] We turn, for a moment, to explore each of these as a context for the remainder of the book.

The fundamental character of illness is the subjective experience that begins when a person detects some bodily symptoms that result in discomfort and/or suffering as well as a profound sense of new limits on their routine daily activity. Pellegrino[2] notes that the person as patient suffers a break in the usual connection between one's self and one's body. In a state of illness, the body stands separately from the self. Instead of the body serving the self, the self must now serve the body. Pellegrino[2,pp. 44–5] refers to this state as an ontological assault and goes on to say:

> This ontological assault is aggravated by the loss of most of the freedoms we identify as peculiarly human. The patient is no longer free to make rational choices among alternatives. He lacks the knowledge and the skills necessary to cure himself or gain relief of pain and suffering . . . Voluntarily or not, the patient is forced to place himself under the power of another person, the health professional, who has the knowledge and the skills which can heal— but also harm. This involuntary need grounds the axiom of vulnerability from which follows the obligations of the physician . . . The state of being ill is therefore a state of *"wounded humanity,"* of a person compromised in his fundamental capacity to deal with his vulnerability. (emphasis added)

It is important to note that to heal the wounded humanity of the patient, the clinician must not only be technically competent but she must also be competent to enter the narrative and private world of the patient.[6]

Confronted with a vulnerable patient,* the health professional makes a profession, i.e. an implicit declaration that she has special knowledge and skills to heal or at least help to do what is in the best interests of the patient, not her own. This act of profession is a moral promise made to the person who is dependent and in need and, hence, who is psychologically and emotionally vulnerable. Under such circumstances, Pellegrino[2,p. 46] notes:

> The relationship between the professional and those he or she serves is characterized by an inequality in which the professional holds the balance of power. All the usual ethical obligations of making and keeping promises apply, but with a difference—the inequality of power poses special obligations on the person who professes. The professional-client relationship is not simply a contract between equals in which each party can negotiate in his own interest, since one part is not free *not* to negotiate.

When the ill patient visits her physician, she co-constructs a narrative or story with the clinician.[5,7–9] This action provides a context to address three questions: What is wrong? What can be done about it? What should be done? While responses to all three questions need to be based on a complex process of

---

* Patient vulnerability is a matter of degree and not difference. It is not the case that patients are either vulnerable or not. Rather, patients who visit their health care provider come to that encounter in a wide range of emotional and psychological suffering, i.e. vulnerability.

narrative exchanges between patient and clinician,[5,10] it is in the consideration of the last question that the patient's interests are paramount and the clinician's full and sensitive elicitation and understanding of them are critical. Consequently, the end of medicine is to exercise a form of clinical judgment that is informed by both scientific and technical expertise as well as a narrative and relationship-centered understanding of the patient.

Thus, what constitutes the internal morality of the medical profession is bounded and contextualized by the nature of illness, the act of profession, and the ends of medicine as a practice in the service of the ill and vulnerable. As we offer the contours of a transformed primary care practice, we along with you, are obliged to continually consider the degree to which various proposed strategies for compassionate and efficient care along with technological applications and financial models for the business elements of practice support the moral relationships between patient and health care professional, as well as among those professionals.

REFERENCES

1 Pellegrino ED. Professionalism, profession and the virtues of the good physician. *Mt Sinai J Med.* 2002; **69**(6): 378–84.

2 Pellegrino ED. Towards a reconstruction of medical morality: the primacy of the act of profession and the fact of illness. *J Med Philos.* 1979; **4**(1): 32–56.

3 Berwick DM. What "patient-centered" should mean: confessions of an extremist. *Health Affairs.* doi: 10.1377/hlthaff.28.4.w555.

4 Rosenthal TC. The Medical Home: growing evidence to support a new approach to primary care. *J Am Board Fam Med.* 2008; **21**(5): 427–40. doi: 10.3122/jabfm.2008.05.070287. 2009 May; **28**(4) w555–6. Available at: www.jabfm.org (accessed October 4, 2009).

5 Engel J, Pethtel L, Zarconi J, Missimi S. *Narrative in Health Care: healing patients, practitioners, profession, and community.* Oxford: Radcliffe Publishing; 2008.

6 Pellegrino ED, Thomasma DC. *A Philosophical Basis of Medical Practice: toward a philosophy and ethics of healing professions.* New York: Oxford University Press; 1981.

7 Greenhalgh T. *What Seems to be the Trouble? Stories in illness and healthcare.* Oxford: Radcliffe Publishing; 2006.

8 Launer J. *Narrative-based Primary Care: a practical guide.* Oxford: Radcliffe Medical Press; 2002.

9 Charon R. *Narrative Medicine: honoring stories of illness.* New York: Oxford University Press; 2006.

10 Stacey RD. *Complexity and Group Process: a radically social understanding of individuals.* New York: Brunner-Routledge; 2003.

CHAPTER 4

The movement toward patient-centered/relationship-centered medical homes

The US may be catching up to other nations in recognizing that primary care must be the foundation of a just, effective, and efficient health care system. This is happening in part because of "natural experiments" by large employers who have found that by providing easy access to primary care (in many cases, by means of worksite clinics), their employees have less time lost from work and improved measures of overall health, while the employers realize significant savings in health care spending, which they can invest in better wages and strategic development initiatives.[1,2] Compare this to the norm for most US employers, who have seen the cost of health care insurance go up by 120% over the past decade, while wages have only kept up with inflation despite significant improvements in worker productivity.[3] Clearly, all that extra production and the associated profits are being devoured by runaway spending on health care. International models of health care delivery and increasing numbers of large employer experiences provide compelling evidence that a highly functional primary care base makes it possible to achieve the Institute for Healthcare Improvement's "triple aim" of improved quality, improved experience of care, and managed costs. Organizations such as the Patient Centered Primary Care Collaborative led by Dr Paul Grundy from IBM[4] are bringing together businesses, insurers, and clinicians to advocate for a primary care based health care system in the US and to showcase emerging models for achieving the triple aim.

In response to staggering health care costs and a belief that basic health care is a right rather than an earned privilege, health care reform efforts in the US may soon provide "insurance for [nearly] all," but there is nothing in the current legislation that directly addresses the cost of care. The experience of Massachusetts, which mandated health insurance coverage and which has achieved a remarkable 96% coverage rate, has seen its health care costs continue to climb,[5] in part because the existing primary care system in the state was not able to absorb the 430 000 additional people who suddenly had insurance. Unable to access a primary care practice, many turn to emergency rooms for routine illnesses, and continue to have no ongoing attention to their hypertension, diabetes, asthma, and other chronic diseases. They have no preventive service delivery—people can't get pap smears in the emergency room, and emergency physicians don't order mammograms or colonoscopies. Repeating Massachusetts on a national scale is a frightening proposition, particularly when one examines the state of readiness of existing primary care offices.

National organizations of PCPs are very clear about what primary care *ought* to be. The American Academy of Family Physicians (AAFP) has articulated an idealized model of practice that would have the following key features:

➤ personal medical home
➤ patient-centered care
➤ team approach to care
➤ elimination of barriers to access
➤ advanced information systems, including a standardized electronic health record (EHR)
➤ redesigned, more functional offices
➤ whole-person orientation
➤ care provided in a community context
➤ focus on quality and safety
➤ enhanced practice finance
➤ defined basket of services.[6]

More recently, the AAFP has joined with the American Academy of Pediatrics, the American College of Physicians, and the American Osteopathic Association to issue joint principles for a "patient-centered medical home" (PCMH):

Personal physician. Each patient has an ongoing relationship with a personal physician trained to provide first contact, continuous and comprehensive care.

Physician directed medical practice. The personal physician leads a team of individuals at the practice level who collectively take responsibility for the ongoing care of patients.

Whole-person orientation. The personal physician is responsible for providing for all the patient's health care needs or taking responsibility for appropriately arranging care with other qualified professionals. This includes care for all stages of life, acute care, chronic care, preventive services, and end-of-life care.

Care is coordinated and/or integrated across all elements of the complex health care system (e.g. subspecialty care, hospitals, home health agencies, nursing homes) and the patient's community (e.g. family, public and private community-based services). Care is facilitated by registries, information technology, health information exchange and other means to assure that patients get the indicated care when and where they need and want it in a culturally and linguistically appropriate manner.

Quality and safety are hallmarks of the medical home:

➤ Practices advocate for their patients to support the attainment of optimal, patient-centered outcomes that are defined by a care planning process driven by a compassionate, robust partnership between physicians, patients, and the patient's family.

➤ Evidence-based medicine and clinical decision-support tools guide decision making.

➤ Physicians in the practice accept accountability for continuous quality improvement through voluntary engagement in performance measurement and improvement.

➤ Patients actively participate in decision making and feedback is sought to ensure patients' expectations are being met.

➤ Information technology is utilized appropriately to support optimal patient care, performance measurement, patient education, and enhanced communication.

➤ Practices go through a voluntary recognition process by an appropriate non-governmental entity to demonstrate that they have the capabilities to provide patient-centered services consistent with the medical-home model.

➤ Patients and families participate in quality-improvement activities at the practice level.

Enhanced access to care is available through systems such as open scheduling, expanded hours and new options for communication between patients, their personal physician, and practice staff.

Payment appropriately recognizes the added value provided to patients who have a patient-centered medical home. The payment structure should be based on the following framework.

➤ It should reflect the value of physician and non-physician staff patient-centered care management work that falls outside of the face-to-face visit.

➤ It should pay for services associated with coordination of care both within a given practice and between consultants, ancillary clinicians, and community resources.

➤ It should support adoption and use of health information technology for quality improvement.

➤ It should support provision of enhanced communication access such as secure email and telephone consultation.

➤ It should recognize the value of physician work associated with remote monitoring of clinical data using technology.

➤ It should allow for separate fee-for-service payments for face-to-face visits. (Payments for care management services that fall outside of the face-to-face visit, as described above, should not result in a reduction in the payments for face-to-face visits.)

➤ It should recognize case-mix differences in the patient population being treated within the practice.

➤ It should allow physicians to share in savings from reduced hospitalizations associated with physician-guided care management in the office setting.

➤ It should allow for additional payments for achieving measurable and continuous quality improvements.[7]

These are wonderful ideals for which to strive, but unfortunately, as in many things, there is a rather large discrepancy between intent and practice. A recent survey of family medicine practices in Virginia indicated that only 1% has established all the elements of the PCMH.[8] Another metric is to apply the standards for the PCMH that derive from the National Council for Quality Assurance (NCQA). These fall into nine categories with a total of 30 elements.

Standards for PCMH[9]

Standard 1: Access and communication

A   Has written standards for patient access and patient communication**

B   **Uses data to show it meets its standards for patient access and communication** **

Standard 2: Patient tracking and registry functions

A   Uses data system for basic patient information (mostly non-clinical data)

B   Has clinical data system with clinical data in searchable data fields

C   Uses the clinical data system

D   **Uses paper or electronic-based charting tools to organize clinical information** **

E   **Uses data to identify important diagnoses and conditions in practice** **

F   Generates lists of patients and reminds patients and clinicians of services needed (population management)

Standard 3: Care management

A **Adopts and implements evidence-based guidelines for three conditions****

B Generates reminders about preventive services for clinicians

C Uses non-physician staff to manage patient care

D Conducts care management, including care plans, assessing progress, addressing barriers

E Coordinates care/follow-up for patients who receive care in inpatient and outpatient facilities

Standard 4: Patient self-management support

A Assesses language preference and other communication barriers

B **Actively supports patient self-management****

Standard 5: Electronic prescribing

A Uses electronic system to write prescriptions

B Has electronic prescription writer with safety checks

C Has electronic prescription writer with cost checks

Standard 6: Test tracking

A **Tracks tests and identifies abnormal results systematically****

B Uses electronic systems to order and retrieve tests and flag duplicate tests

Standard 7: Referral tracking

A **Tracks referrals using paper-based or electronic system****

Standard 8: Performance reporting and improvement

A **Measures clinical and/or service performance by physician or across the practice****

B Survey of patients' care experience

C **Reports performance across the practice or by physician****

D Sets goals and takes action to improve performance

E Produces reports using standardized measures

F Transmits reports with standardized measures electronically to external entities

Standard 9: Advanced electronic communications

A Availability of Interactive Website

B Electronic Patient Identification

C Electronic Care Management Support

****Must Pass Elements**[9]

While criticized for being overly focused on technology and under-focused on continuity, comprehensive care, and narrative care,[10,11] they are nonetheless the measure by which primary care practices will be judged in the context of financial incentives for quality. Practices will be paid differentially on whether they have achieved NCQA Level 1, 2, or 3 PCMH statuses. There seems to be a long way to go when practices are currently measured against these criteria if the state of Virginia is at all typical for the rest of the US: as of October, 2009, only one family medicine practice in Virginia had achieved Level 3 PCMH certification by the NCQA,[11] and there are nearly 1000 family medicine offices in the state.[8]

Is it any surprise, then, that the Massachusetts phenomenon happened, despite the fact that they have more PCPs per population than any other state in the country? The reality is that the majority of primary care practices are inefficient and deliver mediocre care, including the kinds of failures of access and relationship that dominated the reports from those in our earlier study. Can we expect anything different if we provide what Michael Fine has called "coverage without care?"[12] What is lacking in the primary care base of the US health care system is both quantity and quality, that is, we have too few PCPs and too many specialists, and those PCPs we do have are delivering care that they know is far less than ideal. The quantity problem will take years to solve—student interest in primary care must be revitalized, but the lag time between that event and a shift in the US health care workforce is a matter of several years at best. What is urgently needed is a strategy that can be widely applied now, in the context of the current dominant financing mechanism of fee-for-service at rates that reward procedures more than they reward thinking and patient engagement. Furthermore, the quality problem must be framed to include serious work on continuity and comprehensiveness that is provided by health care practitioners who are sensitive to and trained in compassionate and narrative-focused care.[13–15]

It is not just the anticipated tsunami of demand for patient care that creates our sense of urgency, it is also the psychological suffering that is already present for too many patients and their primary care clinicians.[16] Two leaders in the move to improve primary care, Thomas Bodenheimer and Kevin Grumbach, at the Center for Excellence in Primary Care at the University of California, San Francisco, capture this beautifully in their book, *Improving Primary Care: strategies and tools for a better practice.*[17]

BOX 4.1 Primary care problems viewed by physicians and their patients

1   Doctor: I'm too rushed and never have time to do things right.

       Patient: I never get enough time with the doctor.

2   Doctor: It's hard to fit patients into the schedule when they need help, so they are calling and dropping in, creating more work.

       Patient: I can't get an appointment when I need it.

3   Doctor: There's never time to deal with chronic problems. Acute care always comes first.

       Patient: I wish the doctor would explain more about my diabetes.

4   Doctor: It's frustrating trying to get patients to follow my advice.

       Patient: The doctor should stop ordering me around and listen to what I have to say.

5   Doctor: I need clinical information right now, easy to get. How can people expect me to remember everything?

       Patient: I need the doctor to answer my questions with information that I can trust.

6   Doctor: I wish my office would run more smoothly. I'm tired of dealing with personnel problems.

       Patient: The office staff treats me like a number, not like a person.

7   Doctor: I'm always seeing patients of the other doctors. I want to see only my own patients.

       Patient: I have to see a different doctor for each visit.

8   Doctor: Patients are constantly calling my office for advice but no one pays us for answering the phone.

       Patient: I wish I could call my doctor to ask a few questions and save both of us a lot of time. (p. 49; reproduced with permission of the publisher.)[17]

Hear several of the themes that were expressed by our respondents! See how the misery of the patient has its mirror image in the suffering and frustration of the physician, and surely the staff!

Later in their book, Bodenheimer and Grumbach offer a tool for practices to take an unflinching inventory of their processes and how well they are working (Table 4.1), adopted from the Center for Evaluative Sciences at Dartmouth:

TABLE 4.1 Primary care practice: know your processes (core and supporting)

Processes	Works well	Small problem	Real problem	Totally broken	Cannot rate	We're working on it	Source of patient complaint
Answering phones							
Appointment system							
Scheduling procedures							
Order diagnostic testing							
Reporting diagnostic test results							
Prescription renewal							
Making referrals							
Preauthorization for services							
Billing/coding							
Phone advice							
Assignment of patients to your practice							
Orientation of patients to your practice							
New patient work-ups							
Minor procedures							
Education for patients/ families							
Prevention assessment/activities							
Chronic disease management							

They recommend that all those working at the practice fill out this tool and compile the results. They then suggest that processes most in need of repair be worked on by first flowcharting the process and then using this visual display to imagine ways of making the process simpler, more reliable, and more effective. Teams made up of those involved in the process work together to redesign it, using the PDSA (Plan-Do-Study-Act) cycle first articulated by Edward Deming.[18] While we agree that this is a very sound and systematic approach that has worked for some offices, we worry that other offices will look into the mirror of their self-assessment and find most of their processes are either a "real problem," "totally broken," and/or a "source of patient complaint." Might offices that see this picture of themselves react with despair rather than determination? Might they ask, "How can we take time to fix our processes when we are working as hard as we can just to keep up with current demands?"

One response is to seek inspiration from other PCPs that have been in the same emotional place, and have found a way to change the rules of the game, which is the only way of getting out of a catch-22 scenario. The "rules" to which we refer may involve who delivers care and how it is done, how communication occurs within the practice and with patients, and how primary care services are financed. We are aware of a growing number of innovators who are re-energizing primary care in the US, and our next chapter offers some of those stories and the lessons they have for other clinicians and other practices.

REFERENCES

1 Emanuel EJ, Fuchs VR. Who really pays for health care? The myth of "shared responsibility." *JAMA.* 2008 Mar; **299**(9): 1057–9.

2 Zastrow RJ, Quadracci L. Engaging Quad/Graphics employees in the improvement of their health and healthcare. *J Ambul Care Manage.* 2006 Jul–Sep; **29**(3): 225–9.

3 Henry J. Kaiser Family Foundation and Health Research Educational Trust. *Survey of Employer Health Benefits 2009.* Menlo Park, CA, and Chicago, IL: Kaiser Family Foundation and Health Research Educational Trust; 2009. p. 1.

4 Patient Centered Primary Care Collaborative; 2010. Available at: www.pcpcc.net (accessed March 19, 2010).

5 Oliphant J, Geiger K. Lessons from the Massachusetts healthcare experiment. *Los Angeles Times;* Oct 17, 2009.

6 Martin JC, Avant RF, Bowman MA, Bucholtz JR, Dickinson JR, Evans KL, *et al.* The future of family medicine: a collaborative project of the family medicine community. *Ann Fam Med.* 2004 Mar–Apr; **1**(2 Suppl. 1): S3–32.

7 American Academy of Family Physicians, American Academy of Pediatrics, American College of Physicians, American Osteopathic Association. *Joint Principles of the Patient*

Centered Medical Home; February 2007. Available at: www.pcpcc.net/content/joint-principles-patient-centered-medical-home (accessed March 8, 2010).

8 Goldberg DG, Kuzel AJ. Elements of the patient-centered medical home in family practices in Virginia. *Ann Fam Med.* 2009 Jul–Aug; **7**(4): 301–8.

9 National Center for Quality Assurance. *2008 PPC-PCMH Standards and Guidelines* [pdf e-pub]; 2008. Available at: www.ncqa.org/tabid/629/Default.aspx#pcmh (accessed March 8, 2010).

10 Nutting PA, Miller WL, Crabtree BF, Jaen CR, Stewart EE, Stange KC. Initial lessons from the first national demonstration project on practice transformation to a patient-centered medical home. *Ann Fam Med.* 2009 May–Jun; **7**(3): 254–60.

11 Greenawald M. Vinton site achieves Level 3 PCMH status. 2009 Oct 9, 2010 (March 19). Available from www.carilionclinic.org/Carilion/Medical_Home.

12 Fine M, Peters JW. *The Nature of Health: how America lost, and can regain, a basic human value.* Oxford: Radcliffe Publishing; 2007.

13 Frankel RM, Stein T. Getting the most out of the clinical encounter: the four habits model. *J Med Pract Manage.* 2001 Jan–Feb; **16**(4): 184–91.

14 Charon R. *Narrative medicine: honoring the stories of illness.* Oxford and New York: Oxford University Press; 2006.

15 Engel JD, Zarconi J, Pethtel LL, Missimi SA. *Narrative in Health Care: healing patients, practitioners, profession, and community.* Oxford and New York: Radcliffe Publishing; 2008.

16 Linzer M, Manwell LB, Williams ES, Bobula JA, Brown RL, Varkey AB, *et al.* Working conditions in primary care: physician reactions and care quality. *Ann Intern Med.* 2009 Jul; **151**(1): 28–36, W6–9.

17 Bodenheimer T, Grumbach K. *Improving Primary Care: strategies and tools for a better practice.* New York: Lange Medical Books/Mcgraw-Hill; 2007.

18 Deming WE. *Out of the Crisis.* Cambridge, MA: MIT Press; 2000. p. 199.

CHAPTER 5

Stories of success

In contrast to the tales of mediocre to poor performance we heard from the 38 people we interviewed, we have heard stories of primary care practices that are achieving remarkable results. These practices are striving to achieve an ideal model of primary care practice articulated in the "Future of Family Medicine" report.[1] Such a practice has 11 key characteristics:

➤ personal medical home
➤ patient-centered care
➤ team approach to care
➤ elimination of barriers to access
➤ advanced information systems, including a standardized EHR
➤ redesigned, more functional offices
➤ whole-person orientation
➤ care provided in a community context
➤ focus on quality and safety
➤ enhanced practice finance
➤ defined basket of services.

The stories that follow are of practices that have made remarkable progress towards achieving these ideals, despite the fact that they started with a practice model designed to deliver acute care but not chronic care or preventive services, and despite a financing and regulatory environment that creates numerous unreimbursed burdens for PCPs. How did they do it? We will suggest some common themes that seem key to achieving success in these exemplar practices, and then offer a tactical model that we believe can help other primary care practices achieve similar results.

Christine and Tom Sinsky are general internists who practice at the Medical Associates Clinic in Dubuque, Iowa. In an article published in *Family Practice Management*, Christine describes the burdens and feelings that made her decide she and her husband *had* to do things differently:

The primary care visit is becoming increasingly complex and increasingly frustrating for many physicians. For me, the struggles began more than a decade ago. The 1995 version of Medicare's evaluation and management (E/M) documentation guidelines had just been released, with all their complexities and legal consequences. The number of clinical practice guidelines was ballooning, and I felt responsible for complying with each one for each patient. More and more entities were auditing physicians' work, and every month medical journals published yet another article (usually authored by a single-system practitioner) telling primary care specialists what a lousy job we were doing. I found myself spending the majority of my time doing things I didn't find very satisfying: obediently drilling patients through a complete review of systems; frantically searching the chart for labs and past medical information; counting bullet points and getting lost in a maze of coding rules; cajoling patients to reach targets they had no interest in achieving; and then having neither the time nor the energy left to address the concerns that were most important to my patients. In fact, sometimes I barely even looked them in the eye during our visits. After each patient encounter, I would wrack my brain to recall the details of the entire visit and compose an elaborate note that would satisfy lawyers, auditors and anyone else who might look over my shoulder. Generating these notes could take as long as the encounters themselves, and I found myself in the absurd position of spending a substantial portion of my day performing rote, clerical activities. I felt at risk of becoming a guideline-following automaton—a documentation drone. I finally asked myself, "How do I meet all of these guidelines and requirements and still have the energy and emotional reserve to connect with my patients?" I realized that if I was going to survive and enjoy medicine again, I would need to redesign my practice, a 10-physician office operating within a 100-physician multispecialty clinic.[2, p. 28]

Christine and Tom devised a dozen practical strategies that allowed them to recapture the joy of practice and deliver higher quality care.
1 Getting pre-appointment labs so that results could be reviewed at the time of the office visit.
2 Chart preparation by nurses the day before the scheduled visit so that the physician has all needed information such as test results, reports from consultants, and flowsheets for chronic disease management and prevention organized and readily available at the time of the visit.
3 Pre-appointment patient questionnaires that elicit the patient's chief concerns for the visit, elicit a brief review of systems (symptoms), and update

health-related behaviors and family history.

4 Empowering nurses by treating them as partners in caring for the patient, and having them solicit the basics of the patients history, perform standing orders such as immunizations when indicated, and conducting appropriate tests when the patient's condition warrants.

5 Physician preparation by reviewing the assembled information before entering the room and, when appropriate, briefly discussing the patient's needs as discerned by the nurse.

6 Physician presence with the patient, which is possible because so much of what once distracted the physician has been eliminated.

7 Prescription management by having all chronic medications reviewed and prescribed in the context of an annual visit, thereby eliminating most of the phone calls or faxes for prescription renewals that absorb an enormous amount of staff and physician time.

8 Post-appointment order sheet that lists the most commonly ordered labs and investigations and links them with the diagnosis code most commonly associated with them so that staff can quickly enter the order and code.

9 Dictation templates that are mini-scripts for portions of visits that show little variation across patients.

10 Simplified coding rubric that helps ensure that required documentation elements are present in the record and thereby promotes payment for services rendered.

11 Annual exam as an organizing structure, during which prevention, chronic disease management, and medication management are concurrently and coherently addressed.

12 Rapid access scheduling that allows patients to be seen the day they want to be seen, rather than having to wait weeks or months for a non-urgent visit, or be squeezed in for an acute care visit and receive a rushed and perfunctory evaluation.

Christine sums it up by saying:

> Improving office practice is a worthwhile endeavor. Even in the face of complex coding rules, practice guidelines and performance demands, physicians who develop an organized system of information management and workflow and who foster an empowered nursing staff can achieve a productive and satisfying model of practice for patients, staff and themselves. Implementing any of the strategies described here can improve efficiency, but together they can transform your practice.[2,p. 34]

Family physician Peter Anderson of Hilton Family Practice in Newport News, Virginia, was feeling burned out and disheartened, for many of the same reasons listed by Christine Sinsky. Although unaware of the model the Sinskys espoused, he had heard of an internist in Kentucky who was using nurses to obtain and enter the patient's history into the medical record, saving the physician significant time and effort. Peter reasoned that the office visit had four components: Part 1: Data gathering, Part 2: Analysis of data and pertinent physical exam, Part 3: Decision making and development of a plan, Part 4: Implementation of the plan and patient education. Although physicians are taught that historical information is usually the most important and useful part of the patient's data, it is also the most time-consuming aspect of the office visit. He saw that physician-level skills were really only needed for Parts 2 and 3 of his framework, and believed he could train his nurses to do more than they had previously done by taking most of the patient's history and entering it into his practice's electronic medical record. Guided by templates developed by Peter himself, and after several weeks of coaching and practice, Peter's nurses now take the entire history and present that to him after he enters the room and greets his patient. He may add to it a bit, then performs the appropriate physical exam and, with the patient's involvement, states a diagnosis and treatment plan, all of which is entered in the electronic record by his nurse. Meanwhile, another nurse has completed the history for Peter's next patient, and he moves on and repeats the process. He has twice the clinical support staff of most PCPs (as do the Sinskys), but his capacity for care is enormously improved by doing only doctor-level work. He can see many more patients per day in the same time, and his team care approach has significantly improved his practice finances. Peter's collections have increased from $370 000 in 2002, before he implemented team care, to $590 000 in 2007, with a fully implemented team care model. His income and benefits equal approximately 40% of his collections. He sees 540 patients per month, on average, and spends 40–44 hours in practice per week, with five weeks paid time off per year. Equally impressive is the impact that team care has made on measures of care quality. Before he started the team care approach, his outpatient care quality scores such as blood pressure control, diabetes control, and cancer screening for eligible patients were mediocre compared with his peers in a large medical group. His quality scores are now at or near the top relative to his peers, and he earned a perfect score in 2007 on the NCQA Heart Stroke Recognition Program. His patients and staff love the new way of doing things—90% of staff at his office are happy with their job and workplace, and 95% of his patients are happy with their care and likely to return.[3] In Peter's model, patients get detailed attention to all of their needs, with total contact time of 30 minutes with their care team.

Quite a different model for achieving better results has been developed and disseminated by Gordon Moore, a family physician now living in Seattle, Washington. His ideal micropractice model (a solo physician with no staff and very low overhead) has evolved into what he now calls an ideal medical practice (IMP). Moore and his colleague, John Wasson from Dartmouth, ask:

> What do you get when you mix low overhead with high technology and wrap it around an excellent physician-patient relationship? You get an ideal medical practice—a practice model designed to enhance doctor-patient relationships, increase face-to-face time between doctors and patients, reduce physician workloads, instill patients with a sense of responsibility for their health and cut wasted dollars from the entire system. The model encompasses the ideal *micro* practice model, which focuses on optimizing the smallest functional work unit capable of delivering excellent care: the solo doctor, even without any staff. The key principles ideal medical practices pursue are high-quality, patient-centered, collaborative care; unfettered access and continuity; and extreme efficiency.[4,p. 21]

They advocate for practices in which physicians care for perhaps 1000 patients (about half of the norm), and see perhaps 12 patients per day (again, about half the norm), thereby greatly increasing the time they spend with each patient— perhaps an hour for a new patient, and half an hour for an established patient. They call for easy access via phone or email, and have demonstrated financial viability in many markets. Moore and Wasson contrast their "IMP" model with traditional practices.[4,p. 21]

TABLE 5.1 Ideal medical practice versus typical medical practice

Ideal medical practice (IMP)	Typical medical practice
Care is driven by the patient's needs, goals and values	Care is driven by the practice's priorities
Access is 24/7	Access is 9–5
The care team uses technology to the fullest (e.g. electronic health records, email, internet scheduling)	The care team avoids new technology
Patients can see their own physician whenever they choose	Patients must see whoever is available

(*continued*)

Ideal medical practice (IMP)	Typical medical practice
The majority of the office visit is spent with the physician	The majority of the office visit is spent waiting
Overhead is low	Overhead is high
Patients are seen the same day they call the office	Patients typically wait for an appointment
Physicians are able to see fewer patients per day	Physicians must generate high numbers of visits per day to cover overhead
Practices measure themselves regularly	Practices have little or no performance data
Practices are proactive in their care of patients with chronic illness	Practices are reactive in their care of patients with chronic illness
Physicians are satisfied and feel in control	Physicians feel harried and overbooked

Wasson and colleagues have developed a survey tool—HowsYourHealth©—that promotes patient engagement in their own care and provides the care team with a much more complete picture of the patient's self-assessment of their overall function, ability to manage their own care, and confidence in their primary care team and its coordination of their care. It is available to practices and their patients online at no charge,[5] and a simplified version of the online survey is included as Appendix 2. Data to date suggest that the IMPs outperform conventional practices in several patient reported measures that are part of HowsYourHealth. These include overall satisfaction with care, assessment of key care processes, and communication and patient self-management.[6] Wasson's model also creates a remarkable focus on patient-centered care, since IMP practices measure themselves against how their patients answer two simple but powerful questions: Do our patients get exactly the care they want or need, exactly when and how they want or need it? Do our patients feel they are confident in managing their own health care?[5]

What can happen when you change the rules for the way primary care is financed? There are many PCPs who have responded to their stress and burnout by turning to "concierge" medicine. Most of these involve annual fees of between $1500–3000 per person for unlimited access to your PCPs, including house calls when necessary. These physicians typically have panel sizes of about 600, and the hefty fee means that only fairly affluent patients can afford to purchase the service. An alternative has been championed by Chuck Kilo and colleagues at GreenField Health in Portland, Oregon. GreenField still bills insurance companies for office visits, but also charges an annual fee of about $500 per person for unlimited access, including emails and phone calls. Since this removes the incentive for an office visit (typically, the only way PCPs in the US can get paid), it allows the physician and patient to decide when and where and how care is provided. Quoting from their website:

> **Non-office based care is readily available.** To us, service and convenience means we strive to deliver care when and where you want and need it. We do our best to take care of your needs over the phone, and by email if you like, whenever possible. The only time you should be seen in the office is when you want and need to be seen. Of course, a physical examination is often needed to best evaluate a new symptom. However, many routine situations can be handled without an office visit, such as medication adjustments, interpretation of diagnostic tests, and arrangement of consultations with specialists. We can also follow up an existing problem, initiate a family conversation when facing difficult decisions, or answer questions about your care using email or telephone. The choice should be yours, and at GreenField it will be.[7]

Chuck and his colleagues find that most of their day is now spent on the phone with patients or in dialogue via email, with only about a third of the time spent seeing patients in the office. This is one of the reasons that there is no "waiting room" at GreenField Health! Although the data are limited, one of the major insurers with which GreenField interacts tells them that their overall case-mix adjusted cost is about 20% less than other conventional primary care practices.[8]

Some practices have taken it a step further—not depending on health insurance payments at all, but instead charging a flat fee for access and care. Notable among these are Qliance in Seattle, Washington, begun in 1997 by Garrison Bliss,[8] and HealthAccessRI, a consortium of family medicine practices in Rhode Island organized by Michael Fine.[7] These are both "direct medical practice" models for primary care, that is, patients become eligible for care by paying a monthly fee (and, in some cases, a modest co-pay at the time of an office visit). The practices do not bill an insurance company, and thereby eliminate much of the administrative burden and practice costs attached to payment via insurance. This makes access to primary care available to working people without insurance, and improves practice efficiency because physicians and staff don't have to spend time on paperwork related to payment.

These stories of success illustrate several important ideas and strategies. Systematic teamwork takes regularly recurring processes and organizes them so that they are accomplished reliably and efficiently—the Sinskys' pre-visit work and post-visit order sheet and their bundling of preventive care and chronic disease management into an annual visit are elegant examples. Working to the top of one's ability is found in both the Sinsky and Anderson stories, but particularly in Peter's model, where nurses are taking and entering historical data into the medical record. This is both professionally satisfying and a driver of quality improvement, since it allows for an unhurried, comprehensive engagement with the patient and his/her needs. Working to the top of one's ability is also critical for the practice economy, for physician services are what the current dominant financing model is purchasing, and the less time that physicians spend on activities that don't require their expertise, the more time they have to care for patients, which translates into more practice revenue. These practices are able to do today's work today and reduce or eliminate waits and waste by several means. Teams create capacity by both quantity (more horsepower) and synergy (smarter horsepower), allowing for more patient needs to be met in the same time frame. Advanced access scheduling models carefully match supply and demand, eliminating the backlog for both routine and urgent care that is the norm in most US primary care offices. These model practices have the will and the means to measure performance and to collectively work to continuously improve it. They have not let the financing of primary health care in the US get in the way, either by adopting significant efficiencies or by making fee for service, office-visit-based care less relevant or entirely irrelevant.

And they have created and maintained an office culture that gets relationships right—both within the office team and between team members and the patients they serve. As Jody Hoffer Gittell found in the best performing hospitals she studied, these best performing primary care offices have team member relationships characterized by:

➤ shared goals: a wholistic sense of the good of the patient
➤ shared knowledge: the work of others; wholistic knowledge of the patient
➤ mutual respect: value for every team member's role in care.

Communication among team members is:
➤ frequent
➤ timely
➤ accurate
➤ problem solving.[9,p. 53]

Seen differently, one could say that the individuals working in these offices have achieved *narrative and relationship-centered competence*. Such individuals are fully present to those around them and exhibit nonjudgmental acceptance in their interactions. They hear the stories of others fully and can represent them accurately, with sensitivity to nuance and meaning. This is quite different from the clinicians, many of whom we imagine were actors in the stories we heard from our participants, whom patients describe as indifferent, uncaring, or cold. They either lost their narrative competence because of feeling overwhelmed by the relentless pressures of their practice lives, or perhaps because they were never shown that narrative competence matters, and failed to learn and practice these skills during their professional training. "The result is that:

➤ The patient may not tell the whole story
➤ The patient may not ask the most worrisome questions
➤ The patient may not feel that she has been heard
➤ The diagnostic workup may be unfocused and faulty
➤ Clinical care may be marked by 'non-compliance'
➤ A therapeutic relationship may not develop
➤ The clinician may feel professionally dissatisfied."[10,pp. 168–9]

The practices that are models for others have changed the rules by which they operate, and this also makes an enormous difference in how care is designed and delivered. As articulated in *Crossing the Quality Chasm*,[11] the new rules are in sharp contrast with what are typically unexamined assumptions and habits:

TABLE 5.2 Simple rules for the 21st century health care system

Current approach	New rule
Care is based primarily on visits relationships	Care is based on continuous healing
Professional autonomy drives variability	Care is customized according to patient needs and values
Professionals control care	The patient is the source of control
Information is a record	Knowledge is shared and information flows freely
Decision making is based on training and experience	Decision making is evidence based
Do no harm is an individual responsibility	Safety is a system property
Secrecy is necessary	Transparency is necessary
The system reacts to needs	Needs are anticipated
Cost reduction is sought	Waste is continuously decreased
Preference is given to professional roles rather than the system	Cooperation among clinicians is a priority

Clinicians who design and work in offices (and systems) guided by the new rules ensure that *access to care* is timely, continuous with a single clinician/team, guided by patient needs and wants, and is stable and affordable. They create *office environments* that promote healing for all involved, efficiently arranged to minimize steps and promote team communication, yet ensuring patient confidentiality. Patient *registration* is simple and accurate, eliminates redundancy, and promotes respectful communication between staff and patients. *Data gathering* is guided primarily by what matters most to the patient, acknowledging that this will often include narratives of uncertainty and suffering. It is comprehensive in the conventional medical sense, but it also creates an understanding of the patient in context. The means by which these data are obtained is again guided by patient needs and wants, is simple and respectful, and exhibits narrative competence.[10,12,13] *Data organization and representation* is complete, accurate, accessible, relevant, and useful for both patient and clinician. The *plan for achieving and maintaining health* has goals and meaning that are shared by the patient and care team, is guided by patient needs and wants, and is regularly revisited for appropriateness and adequacy. *Access and communication with others that contribute to the plan and its execution* is guided by the primary care team in the interests of the patient, and is coordinated and responsive. The primary care team acts as a *steward of resources*, ensuring that the patient's resources and those of the larger system that finances and delivers care are used efficiently and effectively, being mindful of costs but not avoiding essential care because of cost.

The 38 individuals who told us their stories of avoidable problems and associated harms were probably not among the fortunate few who receive care in places like Medical Associates, Dubuque, Iowa; Hilton Family Practice, Newport News, Virginia; or GreenField Health, Portland, Oregon. Donabedian would say that the disappointing and hurtful outcomes portrayed in the narratives in Chapter 2 are the result of defects in the structures and processes of primary care in the US.[14,15] By structures we mean such things as the composition and responsibilities of the care team or the way the office is laid out, and by processes we mean things like patient registration or ordering and responding to laboratory studies. These lead to defects in safety, efficiency, and reliability. Many have suggested that these problems are not unique to health care, and they believe that the strategies used to solve these problems in other enterprises have relevance to improving health care. We will briefly review two of these strategies and how they have been applied to the redesign of primary care.

Failure modes and effects analysis (FMEA) is an approach to quality improvement that started in the US military, was then adopted by NASA, later by manufacturers, and is now being taken up by service industries, including health care. It looks at processes and determines, by means of experience and conjecture, how a process does or may fail and what consequences those failures have or may have on the end user, such as a patient. A simple example is the way that test results are tracked and responded to in a primary care office. If there is no system to mitigate the risk of an ordered test not being done, or a test result interpreted and responded to, then it is possible that one of those kinds of failures will occur. If the test result is significant, such as a positive screen for breast cancer, then the consequences of delay in diagnosis and treatment can be life-threatening. FMEA starts with identifying the process to study, then assembles a team to conduct an analysis, which in turn involves breaking the process down into its component parts, identifying all possible failure modes, estimating consequences, using this to derive priorities for improvement, then designing, implementing, and evaluating the impact of efforts to improve safety and quality. If one imagines the many processes that are part of primary care, it can be daunting to imagine taking on safety and quality improvement work in an individual office, particularly one that is already at its elastic limit. In an effort to address this barrier, faculty in the Department of Family Medicine at the University at Buffalo have created a simplified version of FMEA which they have successfully used in several primary care offices. Using an anonymous survey, all members of an office assign probability estimates and hazard weights to a list of process failures, and use these to focus on priority issues. In their early work, the investigators found remarkable concordance among physicians, nurses, and office staff, and identified three top priorities: Delays in care due to inappropriate self-treatment by patients, discontinuity of care, and nurse-clinician misunderstandings due to time pressures. The office personnel devised practical strategies to address these problems, and the investigators noted several other patient safety initiatives quite apart from those identified in the survey, and posit that the process of reflection and action had helped create a culture of safety in the participating practices.[16]

Efficiency and reliability are the fundamental goals of the Toyota Production System (TPS) that helped that automobile manufacturer rapidly gain market share (which, ironically, may have contributed to the company's recent quality problems). Not only have other automobile manufacturers adopted TPS with impressive results, but the principles of TPS are being taken up by manufacturers and service deliverers, including health care organizations. TPS strives to deliver to patients the care that they need, when they need it, every time, safely and free of defects, at the lowest possible cost and free of waste.[17] TPS involves mapping processes in order to graphically represent the elements of care processes in detail and thereby make visible the waste that may be present in the form of workarounds or rework that might otherwise be taken for granted as part of the job. It also involves immediate root-cause analysis when a defect (error) does occur, in order to have the most complete and accurate understanding of the basis of the defect, and thereby guide a fix that is more likely to succeed. Finally, front-line workers (in the case of Toyota, people on the assembly line) are intimately involved with the analysis, problem solving, and evaluation. In part because it is a relatively recent addition to the quality improvement tool-box for health care, and in part because it requires some ongoing infrastructure and resources for measurement, reporting, and analysis, TPS has thus far been most fully utilized in the inpatient setting in the US.[18] However, larger health care systems are beginning to make use of it to improve primary health care and are publicizing their work in venues such as the Institute for Healthcare Improvement's meetings on idealized design in outpatient care.[19,20]

While the applications of these ideas and strategies to the improvement of primary care practice design and function have obvious merit, we are concerned that they may be too complex, too reductionistic, and too time consuming for the average practice to contemplate, even if they appreciate them in concept and recognize their potential. We are more inclined to think that FMEA and TPS are properly done by the innovators, and that the resulting models they create can be seen as archetypes for structure and process improvements. Combined with the highly functional models we described earlier, we envision the creation of a menu of options from which existing practices can choose and then person-alize. Tired of the chaos of your practice and the amount of time you spend on activities such as data entry, test tracking, prescription refills, and referrals? Then try the model of team care developed and implemented by Christine and Tom Sinsky, or perhaps you prefer the version created by Peter Anderson. Concerned about the growing number of working uninsured in your community with no access to even basic primary care? Then work with other practices in your community or perhaps with your state chapter of the AAFP to develop a direct practice model in collaboration with Micheal Fine and HealthAccessRI. Or make a complete break with insurance-based payment for your services like Garrison and Erika Bliss at Qliance in Seattle. The point is that individual practices and physicians don't have to each reinvent the wheel in order to get off the hamster wheel on which they now run. It seems to us a better strategy for dissemination is to employ what one of our colleagues calls "R&D"—which in this case stands for "rip-off and duplicate!"

Changing from an existing model to something different is challenging. Physicians are people, and they don't so much resist change as fear it. What if things don't turn out as I hoped? What happens if my practice income falls, rather than remains stable or improves? Will it be possible to go back, or find some way to correct problems that arise? It seems to us that new graduates who as individual entrepreneurs have the maximum freedom for creating a practice that they believe will be a best fit for them and their aspirations, and are in the best place to simply reject the old models of practice and instead choose to adopt one of the exemplar models. The second group of early adopters will likely be people similar to Christine Sinsky or Peter Anderson, who speak about how overwhelmed and demoralized they felt—Peter was actually contemplating leaving the practice of medicine altogether.[3] But rather than abandon their profession, they were determined to find a different way of delivering care to their patients that would re-instill for them the joy of their profession and contribute significantly to improved care for those they serve. Yet we suspect that people like Christine and Peter are in the minority, and that the majority of unhappy PCPs in the US feel stuck and see no way out. They feel no breathing space within which to reflect and consider change, and many of them are at or beyond their elastic reserve. What these physicians and practices need is an incremental approach that does not require much in the way of new knowledge and skills, and that delivers significant early returns with minimal effort. What is required is a stepwise model by which the typical primary care practice in the US can go from overtaxed mediocrity to relaxed, joyful, superior performance that delights their patients and delivers safe, high-quality care. We offer such a model in our next chapter, but we would close this chapter with a summary of our thinking concerning various conceptualizations and practices that have characterized relationships between patients and their physicians.[10] With some notable exceptions,* much current thinking and writing about practice redesign is framed predominantly in terms of economic, political, and technological issues. To be sure, these are important macrosystem considerations. Too often what is lost or devalued in discussions of practice redesign are core microsystem issues concerning the moral nature of relationships between patients and their health care clinicians, as well as among health care provides acting in the service of the suffering.

The nature of the patient–physician relationship has been described from antiquity to modern and postmodern times.[21-26] One thing that is clear in these descriptions of medical practice over time is that there has been a decline in the centrality of mutual relationship and careful attention to the patient's story of illness and suffering, i.e. narrative care.[12,13,25,26] As psychological and structural divides between patients and their physicians have become more pronounced,

---

* Recent work of Thomas Bodenheimer and Kevin Grumbach, both at the Center for Excellence in Primary Care at the University of California, San Francisco, provides a balanced approach to both macrosystem and microsystem issues in primary care. *See* Bodenheimer T and Grumbach K. *Improving Primary Care: strategies and tools for a better practice.* New York: McGraw-Hill; 2007.

there has been a concomitant loss in the appreciation of relationship-centered and narrative practice. The various postmodern critiques of the nature of the patient–physician relationship may be seen as attempts to philosophically and practically reframe the clinical encounter as the core mutually responsive relationship between two people, one of whom seeks attentive compassionate care from the other.

Engel's[27] advocacy for a biopsychosocial model and Balint's[28] creation of the idea of "patient-centered medicine" were early attempts to describe the belief that each person has to be understood and treated as a unique human being. This idea was further developed by Stewart and Brown and their colleagues[29,30] along the lines of a patient-centered clinical method that embraced six separate but related components:

1 pursuing illness as well as the disease experience
2 being sensitive to the whole person
3 cooperatively deciding treatment and management
4 discussing disease prevention and health promotion
5 exploring common ground
6 recognizing structural constraints in the clinical setting, such as time and available resources.

Advocacy for this reframed model of the patient–practitioner relationship tacitly criticized and thus called into sharp relief the characteristics of existing models.

Roter and Hall's work on types of patient–practitioner relationships provides a clear analysis of key variables framing the relational context.[26] They base their conceptualization on the expression of power and dynamics of negotiation between patient and physician. Using the variables of *patient control* and *physician control* each defined at two levels, *low* and *high*, they postulate four types of relationship: default, paternalistic, medical consumerism, and mutuality.

Problems occur when the patient's and physician's expectations of the relationship are in conflict. Communication failures result in dysfunctional and failed relationships that represent frustration and emotional turmoil for both participants. This sets the stage for anger and malpractice.[31] This form of relationship was witnessed in many of the patient stories in Chapter 2.

Paternalistic forms of patient–practitioner relationships are those in which the physician dominates the encounter in all respects, and devalues the patient's illness story. In this model, the patient's role is to seek help and comply with the treatment regimen decided by the physician. The doctor's role is to exercise complete authority in an autonomous society.

Medical consumerism in the US represents relationships in which patients set the agenda and goals of the encounter. This form of relationship has been stimulated by a move from curative to preventive health care, as well as a related and broader social movement that shifts the role of person from patient to consumer.[32] Such a relationship changes the roles of patient and physician by shifting their relative status, decreasing physician authority and increasing patient autonomy. Care is centered on the preferences and values of the patient. Extreme forms of this type of relationship can be misunderstood and misinterpreted as honoring patient-centeredness on the part of some clinicians.

Encounters of mutuality change the social relationship between patient and practitioner. The power in this relationship is balanced and the particulars of each encounter are negotiated between patient and physician. Here the physician actively honors the patient's story and mutually constructs and reconstructs the narrative through a complex process of respectful listening and responding to each other's values, vulnerabilities, strengths, and expertise. There is a search for mutual personhood.

The work of Roter and Hall, along with that of others, foreshadowed the next development in ways of constructing the moral relationship between patient and physician. It was a careful examination of the philosophy and practice of patient-centered care that led the Pew-Fetzer Task Force on Advancing Psychosocial Health Education in 1992 to suggest the next iteration toward a practice of medical care.[33] The group developed an explicitly values-based foundation for the work of health care practitioners, known as *relationship-centered care* (RCC). This model of care is predicated upon four related principles.

1 Health care relationships ought to include characteristics of personhood as well as roles.
2 Health care relationships must recognize the important and central place of affect and emotion.
3 Mutuality is a hallmark of all health care relationships.
4 There is a moral foundation to RCC.

The Institute of Medicine's report, *Crossing the Quality Chasm: a new health system for the 21st century*,[11] affirmed these principles.

Thus, RCC represents the latest development in a series of moves to turn the patient–practitioner relationship from its potentially dehumanizing form within an exclusively framed biomedical model to a form that is sensitive to the subjectivity of both patient and practitioner(s). Finally, we would note that recent work by Lanham, McDaniel, and colleagues,[34] using a complex adaptive systems (CAS) framework moves the idea of relationship to an organizational level. Their work is important in showing how a model of practice relationships based on qualities that support the subjectivity of both patient and physician—trust, mindfulness, respectful interaction, diversity, social/task relatedness, and rich/lean communication—influence practice-level quality outcomes.

With this historical view of relationships between patients and their health care practitioners in mind, we now present an expanded version of the "10-step" approach by which suffering practices can achieve a "patient-centered/relationship-centered medical home" and recapture the joy of serving patients' needs.

REFERENCES

1 Martin JC, Avant RF, Bowman MA, Bucholtz JR, Dickinson JR, Evans KL, *et al*. The future of family medicine: a collaborative project of the family medicine community. *Ann Fam Med*. 2004 Mar–Apr; 2 Suppl. 1: S3–32.

2 Sinsky CA. Improving office practice: working smarter, not harder. *Fam Pract Manag*. 2006 Nov–Dec; **13**(10): 28–34.

3 Anderson P, Halley MD. A new approach to making your doctor-nurse team more productive. *Fam Pract Manag*. 2008 Jul–Aug; **15**(7): 35–40.

4 Moore LG, Wasson JH. The ideal medical practice model: improving efficiency, quality and the doctor-patient relationship. *Fam Pract Manag*. 2007 Sep; **14**(8): 20–4.

5 Ideal Medical Home. Available at: www.idealmedicalhome.org (accessed January 19, 2010).

6 Wasson JH, Anders SG, Moore LG, Ho L, Nelson EC, Godfrey MM, *et al*. Clinical microsystems, part 2. Learning from micro practices about providing patients the care they want and need. *Jt Comm J Qual Patient Saf*. 2008 Aug; **34**(8): 445–52.

7 HealthAccess RI. Rhode Island; 2010. Available at: www.healthaccessri.com (accessed January 15, 2010).

8 Robert Graham Center for Policy Studies in Primary Care. *Primary Care Physicians by State*; 2009. Available at: www.graham-center.org/online/etc/medialib/graham/documents/data-tables/2009/dt001-physicians-state.Par.0001.File.tmp/pc-physicians.pdf (accessed March 19, 2010).

9 Gittell JH. *High Performance Healthcare: using the power of relationships to achieve quality, efficiency and resilience*. New York: McGraw-Hill; 2009.

10 Engel JD, Zarconi J, Pethtel LL, Missimi SA. *Narrative in Health Care: healing patients, practitioners, profession, and community*. Oxford and New York: Radcliffe Publishing; 2008.

11 Committee on Quality of Health Care in America, Institute of Medicine. *Crossing the Quality Chasm: a new health system for the 21st century*. Washington, DC: National Academy Press; 2001.

12 Charon R. *Narrative Medicine: honoring the stories of illness*. Oxford and New York: Oxford University Press; 2006.

13 Greenhalgh T. *What Seems to be the Trouble? Stories in illness and healthcare.* Oxford: Radcliffe Publishing; 2006.

14 Donabedian A. Evaluating the quality of medical care. *Milbank Mem Fund Q.* 1966 Jul; **44**(3): S166–206.

15 Donabedian A. The quality of care. How can it be assessed? *JAMA.* 1988 Sep 23–30; **260**(12): 1743–48.

16 Singh R, Singh A, Taylor JS, Rosenthal T, Singh S, Singh G. Building earning practices with self-empowered teams for improving patient safety. *J Health Man.* 2006 Jan; **8**(1): 91–118.

17 Nowinski CV, Mullner RM. Patient safety: solutions in managed care organizations? *Qual Manag Health Care.* 2006 Jul–Sep; **15**(3): 130–6.

18 Printezis A, Gopalakrishnan M. Current pulse: can a production system reduce medical errors in health care? *Qual Manag Health Care.* 2007 Jul–Sep; **16**(3): 226–38.

19 Clifford C, VanSambeek N, Moard D. Transforming primary care using lean principles. March 23, 2009; 10th Annual International Summit on Redesigning the Clinical Office Practice; Vancouver, BC.

20 Goodman P, McDonald N, Loomis LW, Gutierrez P. Introduction to applying lean principles to clinic flow. March 23, 2009; 10th Annual International Summit on Redesigning the Clinical Office Practice; Vancouver, BC.

21 Szasz TS, Hollender MH. A contribution to the philosophy of medicine; the basic models of the doctor-patient relationship. *AMA Arch Intern Med.* 1956 May; **97**(5): 585–92.

22 Szasz TS, Knoff WF, Hollender MH. The doctor-patient relationship and its historical context. *Am J Psychiatry.* 1958 Dec; **115**(6): 522–8.

23 Lain EP. *Doctor and Patient.* New York: McGraw-Hill; 1969.

24 Shorter E. *Doctors and their Patients: a social history.* Piscataway, NJ: Transaction Publishers; 1991.

25 Roter DL. The enduring and evolving nature of the patient–physician relationship. *Patient Educ Couns.* 2000; **39**: 5–15.

26 Roter DL, Hall JA. *Doctors Talking with Patients/Patients Talking with Doctors: improving communication in medical visits.* 2nd ed. Westport, CT: Praeger; 2006.

27 Engel GL. The need for a new medical model: a challenge for biomedicine. *Science.* 1977 Apr; **196**(4286): 129–36.

28 Balint E. The possibilities of patient-centered medicine. *J R Coll Gen Pract.* 1969 May; **17**(82): 269–76.

29 Stewart M, Brown JB, Weston WW, *et al. Patient-centered Medicine: transforming the clinical method.* 2nd ed. Oxford: Radcliffe Medical Press; 2003.

30 Brown JB, Stewart M, Weston WW, editors. *Challenges and Solutions in Patient-centered Care: a case book.* Oxford: Radcliffe Medical Press; 2002.

31 Levinson W, Roter DL, Mullooly JP, Dull VT, Frankel RM. Physician-patient communication. The relationship with malpractice claims among primary care physicians and surgeons. *JAMA.* 1997 Feb; **277**(7): 553–9.

32 Reeder LG. The patient-client as a consumer: some observations on the changing professional-client relationship. *J Health Soc Behav.* 1972 Dec; **13**(4): 406–12.

33 Pew-Fetzer Task Force on Advancing Psychological Health Education. *Health Professions Education and Relationship-centered Care.* San Francisco, CA: Pew Health Professions Commission; 1994.

34 Lanham HJ, McDaniel RR Jr, Crabtree BF, Miller WL, Stange KC, Tallia AF, *et al.* How improving practice relationships among clinicians and nonclinicians can improve quality in primary care. *Jt Comm J Qual Patient Saf.* 2009 Sep; **35**(9): 457–66.

CHAPTER 6

Ten steps to a patient-centered medical home

STEP ONE: STOP LEAVING MONEY ON THE TABLE

PCPs spend almost all of their patient care time in the office setting, and the vast majority are paid based on the services they deliver to their patients at an office visit. These are billed according to a complex coding system developed in 1995 and revised in 1997 that includes 134 separate "Evaluation and Management" (E/M) codes relevant to primary care, each of which qualifies for potential payment at a rate usually based on some multiple of the payment schedule established by the Centers for Medicare and Medicaid Services (CMS). Once a PCP has established her practice, the vast majority of patients she sees are established (rather than new) patients and their visits (other than for annual checkups) will fall within a group of five E/M codes: 99211, 99212, 99213, 99214, and 99215. Table 6.1 shows the requirements that must be documented in the medical record in order to qualify a visit for one of these codes.

TABLE 6.1 Required elements for most common evaluation and management codes

Elements (need 2 of 3)	99211	99212	99213	99214	99215
History					
History of present illness	Simple problem	1	1	4 (or 2	4 (or 2
Review of systems	that may not		1	chronic)	chronic)
Past/family/social history	need physician			2	10
	evaluation			1	2
Exam* (# systems)		0	2	5	8
Complexity (2/3)					

(*continued*)

Elements (need 2 of 3)	99211	99212	99213	99214	99215
Diagnosis		1	2	3	4
Data		0	2	3	4
Risk		Minimal	Low	Moderate	High

History: location, quality, severity, duration, timing, modifying factors (or status of 3 chronic).

*Exam: 1995 CMS definitions.

Diagnosis: established problem–stable **1**; established problem–worse **2**; new–no work-up **3** (max 3); new problem with work-up **4**.

Data: lab **1**; X-ray **1**; other **1**; discussion with testing MD **1**; decision to review records/history **1**; review old records/history from non-patient source **2**; discuss with another clinician **2**; independent review test **2**.

Risk: minimal: no meds; low: **1** stable problem; moderate: **2** stable problems or prescription med; high: severe side-effects or disease progression, intensive monitoring, severe psychiatric illness, other potential severe or life-threatening illness, do-not-resuscitate.

(Adapted with permission; check with local CMS carrier since there is some variation in interpretation of these guidelines.)

Family physicians in training are taught the rules for documentation and coding, and are exhorted to do so properly in order to be secure in the face of any potential audit, and to get paid for the work they are actually doing. However, one glance at the table above and it is understandable how a typical primary care clinician could get lost in the convoluted requirements for the history, physical exam, and medical decision-making elements that make up the data behind a given code. Yet if one focuses on the "medical decision-making" requirements for the five codes, it becomes clear (at least to practicing family physicians and general internists) that a clear majority of their established patient visits could qualify for the 99214 code. So given that family physicians receive extensive training about coding and reimbursement during residency, and are presumably motivated to be paid for all the work they do, one would expect that a survey of established practicing family physicians would show a distribution similar to Figure 6.1.

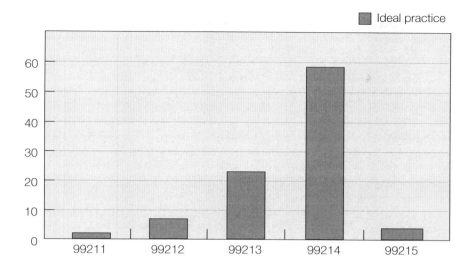

FIGURE 6.1 Ideal practice E/M coding distribution (percent).

In reality, the average distribution that was last gathered from all payer national data in the US (2002) shows the pattern of Figure 6.2.[2]

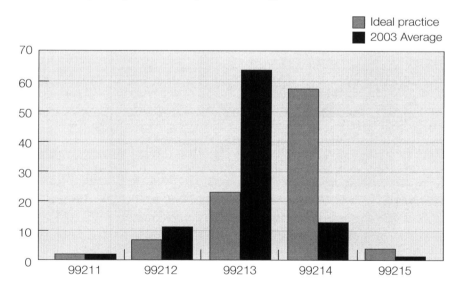

FIGURE 6.2 2003 all payer and ideal practice E/M coding distribution comparison (percent).

And the most recent data for coding distributions for Medicare beneficiaries cared for by family physicians and shown in Figure 6.3 isn't much better, even though these are the patients who are most likely to have multiple controlled chronic diseases, an uncontrolled chronic disease, or problems of uncertain significance such as fatigue, chest pain, shortness of breath, etc. any of which could qualify for a 99214 code.[3]

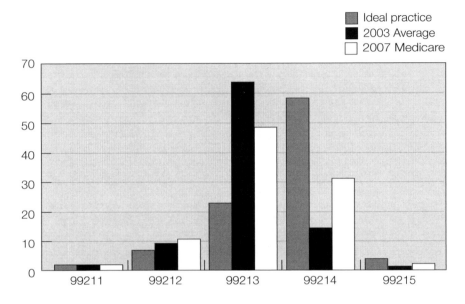

FIGURE 6.3 2007 Medicare, 2003 all payer, and ideal practice E/M coding distribution comparison (percent).

So what does this all matter? It means that the average US family physician is not getting paid for the work she is actually doing—reimbursement that is rightfully hers—because she is either not documenting all the work she does, not coding to reflect her documentation, or some combination of the two. And this is a big deal—the average take home pay for a family physician in the US as of 2008 was $179 682.[4] By not documenting and/or coding properly, the average US family physician is walking away from an additional $50 000–$70 000 in income[5]— up to 39% of an annual income! In talking with practicing family physicians to understand why this is happening, we hear two main reasons: First, the coding rubric is too complex to remember and apply, so coding a 99213 for most visits and 99212 for straightforward visits is safe and easy. Second, many physicians are afraid of being audited (usually by Medicare, but also by commercial insurers), and think that if they have a personal coding pattern that is shifted more to the right, they will invite an audit and the attendant risk for repaying with added penalties. The result of this behavior is to add to the feeling that many PCPs have of being overworked and underpaid. These physicians need to start documenting and coding appropriately to reflect the work they actually do, so they can address the "underpaid" feeling. But how? We believe by making the coding rubric simpler and easier to apply, and by taking heart from hearing how fellow PCPs have survived multiple audits by following the relatively simple steps that ensures that the code matches the record. The best approach we have yet found was published in *Family Practice Management* in an article called "Coding from the bottom up," which points out that coding begins with deciding on the complexity of medical management involved.[6] But rather than try to memorize the entire table of common E/M codes, my approach (AK) in my own practice was to make 99214 my default code unless the visit made me believe that I should code at a lower or higher level, and then I would consult the table to be sure. What I memorized was the medical decision-making criteria for a 99214 visit:

➤ one chronic illness with exacerbation (e.g. poor control of previously controlled diabetes)

➤ two chronic stable illnesses (e.g. hypertension, high cholesterol)

➤ new problem of uncertain diagnosis (e.g. breast lump, back pain)

➤ acute illness with systemic symptoms (e.g. influenza-like illness)

➤ acute complicated injury (e.g. fracture).

There are other elements of the history (e.g. a four-element history of present illness) or physical which are required, but these are also relatively easily remembered, or quickly ascertained with a pocket card. I (AK) asked my partners to read the article and use the same simplifying assumption, and we have shifted our coding distribution from 35% 99214 and 50% 99213 to 65% 99214 and 25% 99213 in a period of a few months. We tracked our coding distribution on a monthly basis for the first several months and made the individual distributions public knowledge among all the physicians in the practice. We focused additional educational efforts on those physicians who seemed to be having difficulty moving their distribution to the right, and now all nine of us show at least 55% 99214s. Our compliance staffs (we are part of a large physician group) tell us that we are still occasionally under-coding, and have no worries should we be audited. So that takes care of the "underpaid" part (or at least it helps). Now, how about the "overworked" feeling? That is taken care of by step two.

STEP TWO: TEAM CARE

It would be tempting to take all the extra revenue generated by step one and use it for that nice vacation, a new car, savings for the kids' college expenses, or a bigger retirement nest egg. However, if PCPs are to make a dent in the problem of inadequate access to their services, rushed office visits, and haphazard attention to preventive services and chronic disease management, they are going to have to invest in more members of the primary health care team, and employ systematic strategies to reduce waste and improve team performance on behalf of the patient. We have referred to some of these team models in Chapter 5, and we wish to elaborate on one of those models here, developed and promulgated by Christine and Tom Sinsky.[7]

The Sinskys have several strategies for improving the quality and efficiency of care. One of these is *pre-appointment labs*. By having the information available at the time of the visit, the patient and physician can review them together and in person, rather than the usual practice of notifying the patient after the patient has left the office, which often involves telephone tag and wastes both the patient's and the physician's time. Another is *chart preparation before the visit*. Because they have adequate staff to support their model of care, a nurse can go through the records of the patients scheduled for the next day and organize the information related to chronic disease management and preventive services. This allows the team to pay systematic attention to these needs, rather than relying on the physician or patient to remember when services are due. It also keeps the physician from having to hunt for medical information—another example of taking non-physician work away. *Pre-appointment questionnaires* allow the patient to write down what they want to cover during the visit, and also provide an updated past, family, and social history, which is important not only for quality of care but also helps support higher service codes (step one). Nurses *work to the top of their license* and obtain historical information, perform symptom-guided testing, administer immunizations according to standing orders, and assist with chronic disease management protocols. *Prescription management* brings chronic medication prescribing into an annual visit, eliminating most of the calls and faxes for refills—often occurring in an asynchronous manner and requiring the same patient's chart to be accessed and the pharmacy responded to several times per year. A *post-appointment order sheet* includes the most commonly ordered labs and other investigations, along with the most typical diagnosis codes associated with those orders. It also includes directions as to when the patient is to be next seen, and the receptionist can place the orders and schedule the appointment.

The typical primary care office employs 0.5–1 medical assistants per physician because these professionals are the least expensive option (compared to licensed practical nurses or registered nurses) and because it comes from a model in which most medical care was for acute, straightforward problems and there were no insurance companies! It made sense then, but it is hopelessly outdated now. In this antiquated model, the "doc does it all," including the following activities:

➤ transcription
➤ documentation
➤ proofreading
➤ paper work
➤ data gathering
➤ data entry
➤ order entry
➤ medication reconciliation
➤ processing prescriptions.[7]

If asked, most PCPs would agree that this is not what they went to medical school and residency to do, and it is one of the aspects of current primary care in the US that is most demoralizing for them. It also represents a huge opportunity cost—no wonder visits are rushed and care is mediocre at best—who has the time to take care of patients the way they deserve when one is being distracted by all these other activities? PCPs can regain the time they want to spend caring for patients by taking a lot of the non-physician work they currently do and give it to somebody else who is competent and who costs far less to employ. Some team care models employ two medical assistants per physician, some have a nurse and a medical assistant, and some have 1.5–2 nurses per physician. Regardless of the particular mix, all of these models use systematic approaches to patient care such as those described above and they can do so because they have the right size and mix of team players and are using processes that are simple and reliable. With this kind of team, patients typically get 30 minutes of attention by *their personal health care team*, and the patient–physician relationship that one of our respondents likened to "farmer–cow" (referring to being herded through the office; *see* Appendix 1) is transformed back to one of a partnership for health that is deeply satisfying to both parties. Other members of the team benefit as well, since instead of merely "rooming" patients and calling in refills, they are involved with ensuring that there is systematic attention to all of every patient's needs and wants, and they see that the team functions at a much higher level because each is working "to the top of his or her license."

Tony Ghaye, a health services researcher from the UK, believes that teams can become re-energized by this success. He says:

[L]earning from success can reaffirm both our capability and capacity for delivering and managing high quality care. Through the practices of team reflection we can learn to notice the successful aspects of our work, no matter how small, and the practical wisdom, within the team, that has led to them. This often goes unnoticed. If recorded in some way, these successes can create positive team memories. These can balance feelings derived from conversations dominated by frustration and a sense of helplessness to change things, anything, for the better.[8,p. 8]

Consulting staff from the Institute for Healthcare Improvement reflect on many years of working with primary care practices, and report that the following features of team care are associated with enhanced patient experiences of care and improved patient outcomes.

➤ "It is clear what is expected of each person at work and he or she has the materials and equipment that are needed to accomplish the role in his or her job. It is easy for care team members to understand and discuss processes of care.

➤ Information for and about the patient's health and wellness is available to the care team when needed (history, diagnoses, laboratory and test results, etc.).

➤ Everyone on the staff is valued, and there is respect and sharing.

➤ Feedback of performance is routine, and there are professional growth opportunities.

➤ Care team members have positive attitudes."

Finally, family medicine investigators Benjamin Crabtree, William Miller, Kurt Stange, and colleagues have demonstrated that practices that pay attention to relationships within the office and form effective teams are more productive, happier places. They offer practical advice on how to go from chaos to teamwork.

BOX 6.1 Tips for building critical relationships

1 **Form an improvement group.** Select members who have different perspectives and opinions. Include practice leadership and representatives from different work groups. Optimal group size is 5–7 members.

2 **Carve out time and space for reflection.** Schedule meetings at least every two weeks. The meetings themselves should last at least 30 minutes. Work from an agenda and make sure meetings begin and end on time. Acknowledge power differentials and strive to make meetings a safe place to voice dissenting opinions.

3 **Set ground rules**
   - Attendance: place a high priority on attending meetings and decide how to bring absent and non-team members up to speed.
   - Participation: every viewpoint is valuable. Emphasize the importance of speaking freely and listening attentively.
   - Interruptions: decide when interruptions will be tolerated and when they won't.
   - Courtesy: listen respectfully; don't interrupt. Hold one conversation at a time.
   - Confidentiality: agree on what kind of information should not be discussed outside the meetings.

4 **Promote active and productive conversations.** Encourage all members to participate fully. Seek out differences of opinion. Search for alternatives that meet the goals of all members, but don't abandon a position simply to avoid conflict. Provide positive feedback on members' accomplishments.

5 **Follow through.** Agree on strategies for implementing, monitoring, and modifying changes that involve all key constituents.[10]

(Reproduced with permission from *Journal of Family Practice*.)

These two steps are hugely important in creating a redesigned primary care office, but they are not sufficient to take full advantage of the potential for primary care to be *"a miracle of modern medicine."*[11] The next step is to take away another barrier to care—outdated scheduling systems.

STEP THREE: RAPID ACCESS SCHEDULING

In an unexamined primary care practice, an unarticulated measure of success is how long it takes to see a physician for a routine visit. The longer it takes, the more popular one must be—how else could the physician's schedule be filled out for two or three months in advance? Problems that arise and which must be taken care of more urgently are either added on to an already full schedule (which further exacerbates the problem of rushed visits for all and increases the risk for both psychological and physical harms to patients), or they are sent to other facilities for care such as "urgi-centers" or emergency rooms, where the patient and her history are not known with the depth of understanding that can exist in a primary care office, and where the lack of certain follow-up results in excessive testing and treatments, with their resulting avoidable costs and risks for harm. So not only is the "long wait—successful practice" a woefully physician-centric perspective, it is also dangerous and costly. But what can one do if one's practice is stuck in this model—hire more physicians? In some cases this is the proper answer, but in most it isn't necessary. What is necessary is exploding the scheduling paradigm so that delays in access to care are eliminated and "today's work gets done today." Such a model was developed in 1998 by Catherine Tantau, a nurse, and Mark Murray, a family physician.[12-14] They called this strategy "open access scheduling" and it is now also known as "advanced access scheduling" or "rapid access scheduling," and we prefer and will use the latter term.

The insight that Tantau and Murray brought to the issue was to see that physicians were *creating* a backlog of two or three months by how they scheduled their patients—they set up a delayed demand for service, and keep repeating that until at some point all appointment slots are filled, with most having been filled one or two months prior to the date of service. It is something like a stream that runs at a constant rate in which one puts a dam—the water backs up, but if the dam isn't too tall, the stream will eventually overflow the dam and continue to run at the same rate down its course. The water behind the dam is an artificial backlog, and so is the two to three month delay for a routine appointment in a PCP office. By this we mean that the demand for primary care services is surprisingly predictable and can be met by matching the supply of primary care services with the demand for same. If you do that every day, you make it possible for patients to see you when they want to—even the same day for a "routine" appointment!

Moving from business as usual to rapid access scheduling requires some pre-work. First, each patient in the practice must be assigned to a PCP. A four-step process can sort out which patient should be linked with which PCP: (1) Patients who have seen only one clinician for all visits are assigned to that clinician. (2) Patients who have seen more than one clinician are assigned to the clinician they have seen most often. (3) The remaining patients who have seen multiple clinicians the same number of times are assigned to the clinician who performed their most recent physical or health check. (4) The remaining patients who have seen multiple clinicians the same number of times but have not had a sentinel exam are assigned to the clinician they saw last.[15] The system isn't perfect, but can be corrected by asking patients regularly who they identify as their PCP.

Second, see if the apparent panel sizes for each clinician are appropriate. As a general rule, family physicians can care for 2000 patients per full-time equivalent (FTE), while general internists can care for 1600 patients (fewer because of the higher proportion of elderly in their panels). (There are more detailed mechanisms to estimate appropriate panel sizes based on age, sex, and visit frequency data.)[15] If some physicians in the group have panels that significantly exceed these targets, it will be difficult for them to provide adequate access and the continuity that ensures, and some of their patients should be invited to transfer their care to a partner who has more apparent capacity.

The next step in creating rapid access scheduling is to standardize and simplify the kinds of appointments that are matched with patient requests for care. In typical practices, each physician has his or her own scheduling rubric, such as 10 minutes for a simple, acute problem, 20 minutes for a follow-up visit, 30 minutes for a complete physical, and 40 minutes for a procedure that takes time, such as excision of a sebaceous cyst. Another physician in that same practice might have different times assigned to these same reasons for visit, making it complicated and confusing for the staff that have to schedule appointments. Furthermore, the reason for visit stated over the phone when an appointment is requested may not be the reason for visit that the patient states when she sees her physician, thereby exploding the careful planning of the physician and staff. Advanced access scheduling calls for making life simpler by having one—or at most two—kind of appointment, and insists that all clinicians in the practice abide by this framework. In my own practice we went from a confusing polyglot system to every appointment gets 20 minutes, unless the physician asks for two slots for a lengthy procedure. Some visits take more than 20 minutes, and some take less, and it tends to even out on most days. Our scheduling people love the new model.

Having identified the PCP for all patients in the practice and right-sized each clinician's panel, and having simplified the kinds of appointment types, it is time to stop creating excessive future demand and to work down the backlog of existing future demand. The first is accomplished by not scheduling patients more than about two weeks out for any needed follow-up, and for patients who are requesting an appointment for routine care to be given that appointment within two weeks of the time they call. The second requires that clinicians not only see the patients that are already on the books, but also the ones that are being scheduled under the new rules. This usually means longer hours (perhaps one or two hours per clinician per day) for a period of one or two months—a psychological hurdle of some significance. Perhaps the best way to overcome this barrier is for clinicians to hear from other offices that have already been through the process and feel their enthusiasm for the new model, and hear how delighted their patients and staff are with the change. In my own office, we made the transition quicker and less painful by doing it during the slowest months of the year (in terms of demand for appointments) and by inconveniencing ourselves a bit by avoiding any vacation or conference time during that period. For readers who want to understand the strategy for changing to advanced access scheduling in more detail, we recommend excellent chapters on the topic by Susan Houck[16] which contain detailed instructions for measuring demand versus capacity and for making a less painful transition to advanced access scheduling. We also recommend the chapter on improving access to primary care in Bodenheimer and Grumbach,[17] which also includes references to other "how-to" and "what difference does it make" resources.

STEP FOUR: INCREASE PATIENT PANEL SIZE

If the typical primary care practice stopped its path of transformation after the first three steps, it would still have created a remarkably improved level of service and performance. Patients could see their personal physician for nearly every visit, and at the time of their choosing. Physicians would have more time to spend with their patients, there would be far better attention to the patient's agenda, to the patient–doctor relationship, and to narrative- and evidence-based care. Finally, measures of preventive services and chronic disease management, and of staff, physician, and patient satisfaction would certainly be greatly improved. However, there is a need to ask practices to do more with this greatly enhanced model of service delivery and care, because there is a growing crisis of access to primary care services in the US that threatens to make a bad situation worse, as we outlined at the beginning of this chapter.

Given that the relative percentage of US physicians that practice in primary care is diminishing each year,[18] and given that the pace and direction of US health care reform that might turn this around is quite uncertain, it seems imperative to ask physicians who have been relieved of the burdens of work that do not require their expertise to devote this newly found time and energy to the care of a few more patients each day, whether in the context of a fee-for-service or a capitated financing system. Assuming the former, which is currently the dominant model in the US, let's say that a family physician who had previously been seeing 20 patients per day were to increase that by four patients per day—two more for each half-day session. This would represent an effective increase in practice capacity of 20%! Given that the average full-time family physician in the US cares for 2000 patients, it would mean an increase in that physician's panel size of 400 more people. The current PCPs workforce for adult care in the US is estimated at 187 000.[19] If half of these would adopt the new model of care and also increase their panel sizes by 20%, it would represent new access to care for an estimated 30 million Americans—a very good start towards providing care as well as coverage. Some of these primary care clinicians might be able to expand their panels even further—team care and advanced access scheduling both introduce powerful efficiencies to the typical office, and anecdotal evidence suggests that full-time family physician panels could be increased to as many as 3000 without diminishing access, quality of care, or patient experience of care.[20] This spectacular growth in primary care capacity would not only provide access for millions who are currently searching for a medical home, but would certainly create huge reductions in health care spending by avoiding unnecessary emergency room visits, avoidable hospitalizations, and duplication of service. Furthermore, a 20% increase in reimbursed practice service delivery would net at least $50 000 in added annual revenue, which is important when considering how to pay for some of the expensive technology we discuss in later steps.

But what of the doctor–patient relationship in this sort of practice? Might we not be risking a return to feeling herded through the visit, and a "farmer–cow" instead of a patient–doctor relationship? Experience with high capacity, efficient practices has shown that a small minority of patients do not like the change, and if given the option, will choose to leave for another primary care clinician that has more physician time in the room. The great majority do not leave, however, and actually rate their overall care experience better than before the practice made the change to an organized team approach.[20] We believe this is so because the care team spends *more* total time with each patient than they did before, because individual patients needs are solicited and responded to, and because no one on the team appears rushed or harried, especially their personal physician. If the physician had heretofore been preoccupied with data gathering, data sorting, and a significant portion of data entry, the new model of team care may allow her to actually spend *more* time engaged with her patients. She can give her full attention to the needs the patient brings to the office, and to what would benefit the patient through systematic delivery of preventive services and chronic disease management.

Based on early reactions to this model from practicing physicians, this step—adding more patients per day—seems to create a psychological problem for some, who say that the first three steps are exciting because they do plausibly suggest a way of enjoying practice again and delivering far better care for patients. Just when they are feeling happy, we ask them to add to their workload and run the risk of feeling stressed again. To them we say that physicians who use a team care model tell us that adding 20% to their patient care volume was easy and that working the same number of hours doing mostly physician-level work is far more satisfying than what they had experienced in the "doc does it all" model of primary care. However, if it helps, and you can afford to add an EMR system without re-opening your practice, set this step aside for awhile until you feel ready.

We have also heard criticism that this model of care enables our broken financing system (fee for service, relative underpayment for primary care services) to be perpetuated, and therefore should be shunned. While we heartily agree that the US health care system needs fundamental reform, the Obama administration's efforts have resulted in a plan to cover more Americans without creating more capacity and with only modest attention to primary care financing. We believe we simply cannot wait for more fundamental reforms when we have models such as the one we espouse that will help create significantly greater access, greater quality of care, happier PCPs (thereby helping attract more students to careers in primary care), and likely lower costs. We ask these critics to think of our model as what William Miller and Carlos Jaén have called "something to do in the meantime" while the US health care system evolves to a more just, effective, and efficient model of care.[21] We also believe that more efficient and effective primary care practices are precisely what are needed when our financing system changes from rewarding doing things to people and instead starts paying clinicians and facilities in organized groups (so-called accountable care organizations) to improve and maintain the health of populations.

STEP FIVE: EXTEND HOURS

At this stage, the practice is humming along nicely, and is at a point of psychological and financial health that it is worth considering another patient-oriented move: to extend hours from the typical 8 or 9 to 5, so that at least on some days the practice is open until 7 or 8 p.m., and on Saturday mornings. This is most workable in the setting of a small group that can envision juggling schedules a bit so that neither physicians nor support staff work more hours per week, just different hours. In some venues, such offices can obtain added reimbursement from commercial insurance companies, allowing them to offer "evening/weekend shift" differentials to both staff and perhaps physicians. Some insurers do this because they realize that access to one's primary care home "after hours" not only improves the quality of care, but also greatly reduces costs by avoiding visits to "urgi-centers" or emergency rooms, whose physicians are more likely to order investigations, at least in part because of no prior knowledge of the patient and no assurance of follow-up. In the absence of differential pay for expanded hours, it may yet be possible to make the case to one's partners on the basis of fostering patient loyalty to the practice and reducing the workload on call—you can go home and count on an uninterrupted night's sleep more often because acute care needs for the day have largely been addressed in the office that same day. Another fallback strategy would be to create linkages with existing "retail clinics" or to create one yourself. If the relationship is functional, these can also serve as after-hours extensions of the medical home. Either option would be a real service to patients with school-age children or work hours that make visits during the day problematic for acute but not life-threatening problems. This step also anticipates changes in the financing of health care towards some form of global capitation, in which so-called accountable care organizations are paid to maintain and enhance the care of a population in the most efficient manner.[22,23] Evening and weekend access to one's medical home had been shown in numerous settings to improve quality and reduce costs,[24] and would appear to be a key strategy for such integrated systems of care and integrated forms of payment.

STEP SIX: PURCHASE AND IMPLEMENT AN EHR

Now that the practice has a more robust cash flow and has created a highly functional team care system in a paper-based environment, it is time to move to an electronic health record (EHR). These systems not only allow practices to essentially eliminate paper records and the attendant expenses associated with space for charts, the charts themselves, and the personnel required to file and retrieve the charts, but they also create the possibility for numerous functions that are not practical in a paper-based environment. These include electronic prescribing, point of care drug choice suggestions, point of care diagnostic and testing suggestions, patient registries (e.g. a list of all patients in the practice with diabetes and indicators of how well you and they are doing on their management of the disease), patient portals (a secure, electronic means for two-way communication with patients—more on this below), and secure linkages with other clinicians of service to your patients (again, more on this later). It seems to us that many physicians are drawn to the power and possibilities of an EHR and invest in a system before they have gotten their paper-based house in order, and we feel this is a serious mistake. Experience has shown that many offices experience great frustrations when they adopt an EHR, including reductions in efficiency and finding holes in system performance that were not apparent at the time of purchase. Indeed, there are a significant portion of practices that abandon their EHR and return to a paper system, having invested tens of thousands of dollars into a failed effort at modernization.[25] These failures are often blamed on poor EHR selection and/or implementation, and it cannot be denied that those are contributing factors in many such cases. However, we believe that another reason for the high levels of frustration and failure is that the typical practice has not done the work to create a more fertile environment in which to plant the electronic seed—they are doing business as usual with relatively low levels of staffing and processes that have waste and inefficiency designed into them.

Yet even a highly functional paper-based office can make mistakes in EHR selection and implementation if they do not approach it in a systematic way in order to avoid common pitfalls. One such approach was developed by Kenneth Adler, a family physician in Tucson, Arizona, who has special expertise in health informatics. He suggests 12 steps for making the decision: (1) Identify the stakeholders and make sure they are involved in the selection process. (2) Clarify what the group's goals are in changing to an electronic system. (3) Write a request for proposal (RFP) to send to vendors that lets them know what you are looking for and asks them to give you critical information about their product and company. (4) Narrow down the list of potential vendors to whom you send an RFP by making sure they have products that work with practices such as yours, and by using published data from user surveys.[26] (5) Narrow down the field of contenders to 3–5 contenders based on the responses to the RFPs. (6) Invite the top contenders to demonstrate their product at your practice site, and have all on the selection team rate the products using a common evaluation form. (7) Check the references provided by the vendors, but also check for users of a given product that were not listed as references, and use a list of key questions during your phone interviews. (8) Select the best two or three products and vendors based on functionality, vendor characteristics, and cost. (9) Visit practices similar to yours that have the products installed and running so you can see how they operate in real life. (10) Select a finalist and a runner-up, in case negotiations don't go well with your first-choice vendor and to provide more negotiating leverage if necessary. (11) Make sure the organization is committed to the product and to the changes and effort required to implement. (12) Negotiate a contract, preferably with the help of an attorney experienced with software contracts.[27]

Adler also offers practical guides for successful implementation. He says that practices that get this right have paid attention to what he calls the "three Ts": teams, tactics, and technology, and his advice is summarized in Table 6.2.

TABLE 6.2 The three Ts of a successful EHR implementation

Team	Tactics	Technology
• Identify one or more EHR champions or don't implement • Make sure your organization's senior executive fully supports the EHR • Use an experienced, skilled project manager • Utilize sound change management principles • Have clear, measurable goals	• Plan, plan, plan • Redesign your workflow • Don't automate processes just because you can; make sure the automation improves something • Design a balanced scanning strategy • Consistently enter key data into your new EHR charts • Get data into the EHR electronically when possible	• Don't scrimp on your IT infrastructure • If you're a small practice, consider an application service clinician (ASP) model • Make sure that your IT personnel do adequate testing • Utilize expert IT advice when it comes to servers and networks

(continued)

Team	Tactics	Technology
• Have clear, measurable goals • Make sure users share your goals • Establish realistic expectations • Don't try to implement an EHR in a dysfunctional organization.	• Utilize a phased implementation • Train, train, train • Be flexible in your documentation strategy and allow individual differences in style • Don't "go live" on a Monday • Lighten your workload when you "go live" and for a short period afterward • Don't underestimate how much time and work is involved in becoming "expert" with an EHR • Pick a vendor with an excellent reputation for support • Utilize "power users" at each site.	• Make sure your servers and interfaces are maintained on a daily basis • Back up your database at least daily • Have a disaster recovery plan and test it.

Reproduced with permission from *Family Practice Management.*[28]

For more detailed information, interested readers can consult the Adler articles summarized above as well as the AAFP's *Center for Health Information Technology*[29] or the American College of Physicians' *Center for Practice Improvement and Innovation health information technology section.*[30]

STEP SEVEN: START DOING POPULATION QUALITY CARE WORK

Five steps back, you created a health care team to systematically address the acute care, chronic care, and preventive care needs of your patients. When designed and implemented properly, this team care approach can vastly improve the quality of care patients receive across those three categories of need for two basic reasons: adequate human resources, and a systematic approach to engaging patients and covering all their wants and needs. It has been estimated that for the typical family physician caring for 2500 patients, it would take 18 hours of every work day to deliver all chronic care and preventive care services.[31,32] This is simply not feasible for an individual physician, but it is entirely possible for a team of health professionals, and much of the work can and should be done by someone other than a physician. What the team is doing is planned care—one of the two central features of the so-called Chronic Care Model developed by Ed Wagner and colleagues at the Group Health Cooperative of Puget Sound.[33] The other central feature of this model is population care, and it is here that your EHR can be of enormous help. Population care refers to an understanding of the entire cohort of patients under your care, designing systems of care that address their needs, employing metrics of their care, and evaluating the results at a population level. It is impractical to imagine a physician in a paper-based system to be able to answer questions such as, "How many people with hypertension do I have in my practice, and how many of them have their blood pressure under good control?", or "How many of my patients are eligible for colorectal cancer screening, and how many of those are up to date with their screening?" EHRs that have a well-designed registry function (and many do not!) can answer those questions quickly and easily. It is important to understand, however, that if you have been doing a good job taking care of the acute, chronic, and preventive care needs of the patients you see on a regular basis, you will not find there is a lot of work to do to take care of those that haven't had contact with the practice in awhile. Recall the model practice in Dubuque, Iowa run by Christine and Tom Sinsky—when they purchased their EHR and turned on the registry function, they found that fewer than 10% of their patients who were eligible for colorectal cancer screening had not had it performed.[34] Compare this to the 50% of people not up to date on this screening in a typical practice,[35] and you can appreciate the power of systematic, one at a time care.

Identifying your patients with similar needs via the registry function of your EHR also allows you to consider an approach to their care using group visits. A common example is to invite your patients who have diabetes to come together to talk about their individual concerns regarding adhering to a diet or exercise program, using their oral medications, employing insulin regimens, or monitoring their blood sugars. The benefit of group visits are many: efficient use of office resources since 8–12 people can receive instruction at the same time (and clinicians can bill for this service for each person in the group, albeit at a low level such as 99212), but more importantly, it provides a place for a small community of people with common needs and concerns to come together and to be a resource for one another. The temptation for clinicians is to be in the role of expert, but the most effective groups are ones in which most clinical questions are answered by group members, with backup from the medical staff, since this is consistent with the ideal of patient self-management and efficacy. For those who are interested in learning more about group visits, consult the relevant sections in the books by Houck[16] and by Bodenheimer and Grumbach.[17]

STEP EIGHT: GET A PATIENT PORTAL

A patient portal is a secure, internet-based mechanism for two-way communication between patients and clinicians. Although some email systems allow for encryption, many patients and physicians are reluctant to use these systems because of security concerns. Since patient portals use passwords and encryption, they provide the same level of security as is afforded by online banking. Major functions of portals include messaging (thereby eliminating phone tag and waiting on hold for staff to answer a call and take a message), access to one's own record (a personal health record), requests for appointments, making payments online, and even providing a detailed medical history in advance of the office visit using tools such as *Instant Medical History*.[36] Some practices also offer "e-visits" when the nature of the service does not require a physical exam, and in some communities, these services are paid for by insurance companies. Since the vast majority of adult Americans now have internet access, providing your patients with this option can be a time-saver for you, for your staff, and for your patients.

Family physician, educator, and futurist Joseph Scherger takes it a step further, and says that the internet and patient portals will literally transform the way care is delivered, and who is in charge:

> The internet makes it possible to give patients more control over their care and challenges the concept of physician-directed care. When patients have their personal health records connected to their chosen clinicians of care through Web-based personal medical homes, what is to stop them from coordinating some of their own care? Physicians who think they will direct patient care in the future might reflect on what has happened to personal bankers, stockbrokers, and travel agents.[37,p. 286]

He goes on to say that this model is entirely consistent with Wagner's Chronic Care Model,[33] which presupposes a partnership between patient and health care team.

> The relationship is symmetric, with the control of care equally shared. Patients are asked to become experts themselves, to develop an understanding of their chronic illnesses that matches or perhaps exceeds that of their physician. With the internet, all knowledge becomes available for free, and learning happens rapidly. Patients, supported by their families and friends, only have their own problems to learn about.[37,p. 286]

There is mounting evidence that patients who depend on themselves and their friends and family for chronic disease management with the support of a responsive health care team do better than those cared for in a model in which they depend upon the physician, who is "in charge."[38-41]

STEP NINE: GET CONNECTED TO OTHER CLINICIANS

Another powerful potential function of the EHR is the ability to communicate securely and electronically with other sites and providers of care, including pharmacies, diagnostic centers, specialists, hospitals, and social service agencies. The major practical obstacles to this connectivity are many, including interoperability of systems, competition among health care systems in a given locale, and lack of financial incentives for their implementation and maintenance. For this reason, they are most developed and functional in those places where an integrated health care system with aligned financial incentives is already in place, such as the Geisinger Health System in rural Pennsylvania[42] or the collaborative among nonprofit organizations that exists in Grand Junction, Colorado.[43] Both of these locations show quality scores that lead the nation and Grand Junction, in particular, has some of the lowest costs for health care in the US.[43] The factors contributing to this level of performance versus cost go beyond just the electronic inter-linkage, but it would not be possible for such organizations and collaboratives to achieve such impressive results if they did not have the ability to send and receive information electronically, and to develop a searchable database of all episodes of care. Other health care organizations and the federal government are recognizing the potential of such networks and are investing in their establishment.[44,45] Even in the absence of a fully developed network, individual practices can obtain free software to implement electronic prescribing, and the best of these programs have been shown to reduce medication-related errors and lower overall medication costs.[46] Virtually all chain pharmacies in the US now can accept electronic prescriptions, and independent pharmacies are rapidly catching up.[47] The CMS has created both a carrot and a stick to incentivize e-prescribing—participating practices will receive additional payments for the next few years and nonparticipating practices will see their Medicare payments reduced slightly. Obtaining an interface that allows diagnostic centers such as labs and imaging centers to send reports directly to your EHR reduces staff data entry time, and may be available at no cost to your practice if the vendor of the diagnostic services sees it as in their interest to keep you as a customer.

STEP TEN: FOCUS ON COSTLIEST PATIENTS

Even in an integrated system with electronic interfaces and aligned financial incentives, there will be a small subpopulation of patients who generate very large health care expenditures. Data from the Kaiser Health Care System in California, for example, shows that 1% of their patients generate one-third of health care expenditures, and that 10% generate two-thirds of costs.[48] This pattern is actually widespread across most settings and payers, and is usually due to inadequate coordination and continuity of care (even when both are available) and inadequate attentions to psychosocial needs that are helping create some of the demand for medical services. Several years ago, a group of pediatricians in the state of North Carolina partnered with state government and introduced a program to identify and better serve the needs of these most costly of patients. They created collaboratives of primary care practices in several regions and provided them with new resource to hire case managers who could proactively work with the most needy patients and link them more effectively to primary care, mental health care, and social services. Independent audits of the results show that this program is saving the state hundreds of millions of dollars annually compared to projected costs of "business as usual" care.[49] The Geisinger Health System has employed an analogous strategy to work with the most costly Medicare beneficiaries for which they care. They have hired nurses to embed into existing primary care practices and have asked them to create a working relationship with the costliest patients as well as with the primary care team and identify ways that they can help better meet the needs of these patients. This effort has had remarkable success in the first 18 months of operation—showing a return on investment of 250%,[50] and the Johns Hopkins Health System has also seen impressive results from a similar program.[51]

Such programs have moral content at the individual and societal level. Patients who have access to continuous, coordinated care but don't avail themselves of that care and its benefits suffer in ways that can be avoided, but they don't have the personal resources to take advantage of what is available to them, and require some sort of active outreach to become engaged with appropriate medical and social resources. The reduction in spending that results from these programs means that more people can have access to care, and those monies that would otherwise have been spent on very costly medical care can be used for other social goods such as educational opportunity, food security, and personal security. We learned recently that the Geisinger Health System has been so helpful in holding down health care costs for one of the Pennsylvania counties it serves that the county used those savings to give their teachers a net raise of $7000 over the past three years.[50]

ESSENTIALS FOR THE JOURNEY

This progression seems simple, and many will say that practice transformation is far more difficult than this framework would suggest. Some say that true transformation to a PCMH requires a fundamental rethinking of what it means to take care of patients, of roles and responsibilities, and of the financing systems that reward procedures far more than the work of trying to keep people healthy. While we acknowledge the obstacles to transformation at micro- and macro-system levels, we believe that the greatest obstacles are the sense that it just isn't possible to make things better in primary care without an external intervention that includes a lot of new capital. This 10-step model is meant to challenge that assumption, and offer hope and a way forward for the typical family medicine or general internal medicine practice in the US, regardless of how and whether health care reform unfolds. If this model is to work, we see four keys to success.

First, family physicians must get out of the 99213 rut that keeps them from the income that is rightfully theirs, and that in turn leads them to stick with staffing models that virtually guarantee performance mediocrity and staff/physician/patient dissatisfaction. Primary care residents in training are exhorted to code properly and given feedback on how it will affect their financial well-being in practice, yet this problem has persisted despite the instruction and despite the relatively low salaries of PCPs. This is probably true for two reasons: a coding rule book that, at first glance, appears overly complex and difficult to recall and apply, and the specter of audit, particularly from Medicare. We have tried to show that the coding rubric can be greatly simplified by focusing on 99214 as the default code for an established patient, and experience in several practices has demonstrated that the coding distribution can shift quickly and with relatively little time spent on instruction, but it is important to use regular reminders and feedback. The fear of audit may be best addressed by knowing that one's peers have shifted their coding distribution to higher levels and have survived audits unscathed. We have brought such physicians to groups of their peers in an effort to create more confidence. Another strategy might be to have a professional coder audit the performance of the physicians in a group during the process of change. Larger networks of physicians typically already employ such experts, and smaller offices can purchase the service. One of us (AK) practices in a large multispecialty group, and the compliance experts from his health system say that his group is still occasionally under-coding, despite a distribution in which two-thirds of established patient visits are coded as 99214.

Second, family physicians will need to allow their innate orientation toward relationships (one of the reasons they chose their specialty) to become as evident in the relationships they have with their colleagues and staff. We believe that by taking the first step we describe above, the physicians will become less concerned about practice and personal finances (a very basic issue!) and be more able to be present to those with whom they work every day. Mindfully engaging all members of the team on how they can function better as a collective will need more than just attention by the physicians, it will also take time—there is no cheap and easy way to avoid what gets done in team meetings. Hence the importance of not leaving money on the table, so that the practice owners have some financial "breathing space." Another skill that might have to be learned and practiced is the ability to handle conflict constructively. Groups in which everyone sees things the same way are not groups that are likely to best discern external threats and opportunities, nor internal strengths and weaknesses. But groups in which differing views lead to defense and distance are also doomed to underperform. Successful groups can have "crucial conversations" in which the stakes are high, emotions are high, and opinions differ. Parties to these conversations stay in dialogue and resolve the conflict by attending to the other's safety needs—one more example of how by giving we receive. Because this is such an important aspect of healthy office cultures, those who are in power positions in the office would do well to read "Crucial Conversations"[52] and ask others to hold up a mirror so that they can learn how they unknowingly make others feel less safe, and thereby keep crucial conversations from happening. Members of practices can also benefit from systematic and sustained training in narrative reflective practices such as those described by Ghaye,[8] Johns,[53] and Engel, Zarconi, Pethtel, and Missimi.[54] And the leaders of practices would do well to consider the call to "quiet leadership" from Ghaye, who says such people make teams work well because they have the following qualities:

 1 good learners—they change themselves, not just others
 2 value driven—they are concerned about what the team stands for
 3 reflect on patterns of power—they encourage a culture of questioning
 4 good readers—they want ideas from everywhere
 5 develop "alongsidedness," not leader–follower relationships
 6 promote self-organized team-working
 7 not thick- but thin-skinned (emotional awareness)
 8 appreciate that little things mean a great deal
 9 resistant to over-responsibility and under-responsibility
10 have a quality of mystique (quietly, low-profile).[8,pp. 204–7]

Third, payers must welcome and support this development of primary care, because it will come with a greater proportion of the health care dollar being spent on primary care services, and less on diagnostic and specialty care services.

There is risk of pushback if the overall picture is not at least cost-neutral, and there are recent examples of insurers using audits, downcoding, and changing reimbursement rates (*"blending"*) in response to shifts in E/M codes by PCPs towards higher codes.[55] Improvements in prevention compare very well to chronic disease management when using a metric of cost per quality-adjusted life year (QALY), even though they may seem to add to the expense of care when they are delivered to all eligible patients, instead of the subset that currently receive them in the US. Moreover, Steve Woolf has pointed out that

> [a]rguing that prevention and disease care are equally cost-effective encounters a more fundamental problem: preventing sickness has value in human terms that econometrics cannot capture. Even if prevention and treatment cost the same per QALY, patients prefer the former to avoid the ordeal of illness. Other societal benefits of improved health—e.g. workforce productivity and corporate competitiveness, and the ripple effects these trends bring to households, education, crime, and other societal outcomes—are among the intangibles that typically go unmeasured in cost-effectiveness studies.[56]

Improvements in chronic disease management are more likely to show both short- and long-term reductions in health care spending, as emergency room visits and hospitalizations are prevented by better attention to conditions like diabetes, asthma, COPD, coronary artery disease, and congestive heart failure. The Patient Centered Primary Care Collaborative recently commissioned a review of the evidence of the impact of PCMH demonstration projects across the US, and they drew two important conclusions:

➤ Quality of care, patient experiences, care coordination, and access are demonstrably better.
➤ Investments to strengthen primary care result within a relatively short time in reductions in emergency department visits and inpatient hospitalizations that produce savings in total costs. These savings at a minimum offset the new investments in primary care in a cost-neutral manner, and in many cases appear to produce a reduction in total costs per patient.[49,p. 1]

Fourth, it seems important for transformation to occur in the context of "communities of practice"—groups of clinicians from different offices who share common interests and needs and who come together to share best practices, solve one another's problems, and generate innovation.[57] Some of these groups form spontaneously at the local level, while others are facilitated by means of common ownership or within the context of an already existing organization at the local of state level, such as state chapters of the AAFP. The Virginia Academy of Family Physicians (VAFP) has begun to be such a vehicle for this activity. Over the past few years, the twice annual meetings have evolved to include not only conventional continuing medical education (such as new developments in the treatment of common diseases), but also presentations by local peers and outside leaders on how practices can redesign themselves and achieve improved results. As of this writing, the VAFP plans to bring this focus to regional chapter meetings and to create additional times and places for more in-depth training and discussion of many of the steps described earlier. Phoenix family physician Scott Endsley has a wonderful summary of what communities of practice can do for family medicine and how they can be formed and sustained. In his overview, he offers a hypothetical welcome to a new group member:

> Welcome to our group! Let us tell you what we do. As you know, we are family physicians from the community who meet here each month to talk about what we are doing in our practices. We discuss common issues and share ideas and approaches to making our practices more efficient and effective. In addition to our monthly meetings, we communicate with each other through an email discussion list that one of our members started. He also started a Web site for the group that allows us to post questions, ideas or practice tools. Our goal is to be more competitive with the large, hospital-owned primary care network in our community by putting our heads together, sharing what we know and sometimes testing new ideas out together. We have recently started pooling data from each of our practices to identify our opportunities for improvement.
>
> One of the members of our group has been participating in a chronic-disease collaborative where he works with other PCPs to find new ways of improving care for patients with diabetes and asthma. At one of our recent meetings, he shared with us some of the tools he had come across in his collaborative workchart-tracking tools, patient-education materials and disease-registry software.
>
> Another one of our members is particularly interested in financial-incentive programs for family physicians and recently attended an AAFP seminar on the topic. He will be talking with us today about pay-for-performance programs in our community. Also, the medical director for one of our local health plans will be here to explain what his plan's new physician incentive program is and how we might participate.
>
> We are pleased that you are joining our community. We look forward to

learning from you, working on problems together and improving how we practice family medicine.[58]

In addition to these local and regional efforts, the AAFP and the American College of Physicians (ACP) have numerous resources for practice redesign available to their members, and much of it is in the public domain as well. The AAFP has also invested in a national demonstration project on practice redesign known as the TransforMED project,[59] and published lessons learned in the *Annals of Family Medicine* in the Summer of 2010.[60] TransforMED is now organized to provide a variety of means whereby practices can obtain consultation, coaching, or facilitation.[59] Such sustained national efforts can facilitate and accelerate the work of local communities of practice, and some of the best ideas and strategies from local communities can find their way to a national audience.

It should be obvious that transformed offices will directly address most of the avoidable problems and associated harms we heard in the stories of our respondents: problems with phone communication, delays in getting appointments, lengthy stays in the "waiting room," rushed visits that don't address patient wishes, much less needs, and the attendant sense of dehumanization. It is plausible that team care and health information technology will also reduce the technical errors we heard about and that have been described in other studies[61,62] such as mistakes in diagnosis and treatment.[63,64] So there are compelling moral, practical, and economic arguments for transforming primary care practices. But as medical educators we offer one more reason why we must do this transformation work now: we need to attract more students into the primary care specialties in the US (particularly family medicine and general internal medicine) if we hope to avoid Michael Fine's "coverage without care" scenario.[65] Study after study has shown that the most important influence on a medical student's decision to choose a primary care career is the experience they have in a community-based practice.[66,67] Therefore, we feel compelled to accelerate the pace of practice transformation in US primary care offices so that every student will see for themselves what is possible—a practice in which a team delivers care that delights the patient and improves that person's life in tangible and subtle ways, a patient–physician relationship that endures and deepens with time, and a level of compensation that removes all thought of considering another specialty just because it pays far better. When we achieve this reality—and we have the tools to do so right now [68,69]—we will shift the US physician workforce back to a point of balance, and at the same time greatly improve access, quality, and efficiency of resource utilization. The economic, moral, psychological and opportunity costs of business as usual are unacceptable and avoidable. It is time to get started.

REFERENCES

1 Sinsky CA. *Coding Made Simple: a case based approach*. Presentation to the Society of General Internal Medicine. Sep 29, 2006.

2 Medical Group Management Association. *Coding Profile Sourcebook: 2004 report based on 2003 and 2002 data*. Englewood, CO: Medical Group Management Association; 2004.

3 Centers for Medicare and Medicaid Services. *Medicare Part B Physician/Supplier National Data: Calendar Year 2007*; 2008. Available at: www.cms.hhs.gov/MedicareFeeforSvcPartsAB/Downloads/Specialty07.pdf (accessed March 30, 2010).

4 American Academy of Family Physicians. *Median Income of Physicians by Specialty, 2008*; 2009. Available at: www.aafp.org/online/etc/medialib/aafp_org/documents/press/charts-and-graphs/median-income-by-specialty.Par.0001.File.tmp/MedianIncome2008FINAL.pdf (accessed April 6, 2010).

5 Kuzel AJ. Ten steps to a patient-centered medical home. *Fam Pract Manag*. 2009 Nov–Dec; **16**(6): 18.

6 Weida TJ, O'Gurek DT. Coding from the bottom up. *Fam Pract Manag*. 2008 Nov–Dec; **15**(9): 22–5.

7 Sinsky CA. Improving office practice: working smarter, not harder. *Fam Pract Manag*. 2006 Nov–Dec; **13**(10): 28–34.

8 Ghaye T. *Developing the Reflective Healthcare Team*. Malden, MA: Wiley-Blackwell; 2006.

9 Sevin C, Moore G, Shepherd J, Jacobs T, Hupke C. Transforming care teams to provide the best possible patient-centered, collaborative care. *J Ambul Care Manage*. 2009 Jan–Mar; **32**(1): 24–31.

10 Crabtree B, Miller W, McDaniel R, Strange K, Nutting P, Jan C. A survivor's guide for primary care physicians. *J Fam Pract*. 2009; **58**(8): E1.

11 John Stoeckle Center for Primary Care Innovation. *Primary Care: a miracle of modern medicine*; 2006. Available at: www.massgeneral.org/stoecklecenter/assets/pdf/brochure_miracle.pdf (accessed March 19, 2010).

12 Murray M, Tantau C. Must patients wait? *Jt Comm J Qual Improv*. 1998 Aug; **24**(8): 423–5.

13 Murray M, Tantau C. Redefining open access to primary care. *Manag Care Q*. 1999; **7**(3): 45–55.

14 Murray M, Tantau C. Same-day appointments: exploding the access paradigm. *Fam Pract Manag*. 2000 Sep; **7**(8): 45–50.

15 Murray M, Davies M, Boushon B. Panel size: how many patients can one doctor manage? *Fam Pract Manag*. 2007 Apr; **14**(4): 44–51.

16 Houck S. *What Works: effective tools and case studies to improve clinical office practice*. Boulder, CO: Health Press Publishing; 2004.

17 Bodenheimer T, Grumbach K. *Improving Primary Care: strategies and tools for a better practice*. New York: Lange Medical Books/Mcgraw-Hill; 2007.

18 Salsberg E, Rockey PH, Rivers KL, Brotherton SE, Jackson GR. US residency training before and after the 1997 Balanced Budget Act. *JAMA*. 2008 Sep; **300**(10): 1174–80.

19 Robert Graham Center for Policy Studies in Primary Care. *Primary Care Physicians by State*;

2009. Available at: www.graham-center.org/online/etc/medialib/graham/documents/data-tables/2009/dt001-physicians-state.Par.0001.File.tmp/pc-physicians.pdf (accessed March 19, 2010).

20 Anderson P, Halley MD. A new approach to making your doctor-nurse team more productive. *Fam Pract Manag.* 2008 Jul–Aug; **15**(7): 35–40.

21 Miller W, Jaén C. Personal communication; February 18, 2010.

22 Dove JT, Weaver WD, Lewin J. Health care delivery system reform: accountable care organizations. *J Am Coll Cardiol.* 2009 Sep; **54**(11): 985–8.

23 Larson EB. Group Health Cooperative: one coverage-and-delivery model for accountable care. *N Engl J Med.* 2009 Oct; **361**(17): 1620–2.

24 Abrams M. *Creating Value: expanded access to primary care*; 2010. Available at: www.pcpcc.net/files/abrams__march_30_2010_ppt.ppt (accessed April 6, 2010).

25 Chambliss ML, Rasco T, Clark RD, Gardner JP. The mini electronic medical record: a low-cost, low-risk partial solution. *J Fam Pract.* 2001 Dec; **50**(12): 1063–5.

26 Edsall RL, Adler KG. The 2009 EHR user satisfaction survey: report from 2 012 family physicians. *Fam Pract Manag.* 2009 Nov–Dec; **16**(6): 10.

27 Adler KG. How to select an electronic health record system. *Fam Pract Manag.* 2005 Feb; **12**(2): 55–62.

28 Adler KG. How to successfully navigate your EHR implementation. *Fam Pract Manag.* 2007 Feb; **14**(2): 33–9.

29 American Academy of Family Physicians. *Center for Health Information Technology*; 2010. Available at: www.centerforhit.org/online/chit/home.html (accessed March 19, 2010).

30 American College of Physicians. *Center for Practice Improvement and Innovation: health information technology section*; 2010. Available at: www.acponline.org/running_practice/technology (accessed March 19, 2010).

31 Yarnall KS, Pollak KI, Ostbye T, Krause KM, Michener JL. Primary care: is there enough time for prevention? *Am J Public Health.* 2003 Apr; **93**(4): 635–41.

32 Ostbye T, Yarnall KS, Krause KM, Pollak KI, Gradison M, Michener JL. Is there time for management of patients with chronic diseases in primary care? *Ann Fam Med.* 2005 May–Jun; **3**(3): 209–14.

33 Wagner EH. Meeting the needs of chronically ill people. *BMJ.* 2001 Oct; **323**(7319): 945–6.

34 Sinsky CA. *Personal Communication re CRC Screening.* 2009 March 24.

35 Woolf SH, Jones RM, Rothemich SF, Krist A. The priority is screening, not colonoscopy. *Am J Public Health.* 2009 Dec; **99**(12): 2117–8; author reply 2118.

36 Primetime Medical Software. *Instant Medical History*; 2010. Available at: www.medicalhistory.com/home/index.asp (accessed March 19, 2010).

37 Scherger JE. Future vision: is family medicine ready for patient-directed care? *Fam Med.* 2009 Apr; **41**(4): 285–8.

38 Bodenheimer T, Wagner EH, Grumbach K. Improving primary care for patients with chronic illness. *JAMA.* 2002 Oct; **288**(14): 1775–9.

39 Bodenheimer T, Wagner EH, Grumbach K. Improving primary care for patients with chronic illness: the chronic care model, part 2. *JAMA*. 2002 Oct; **288**(15): 1909–14.

40 Bodenheimer T, Lorig K, Holman H, Grumbach K. Patient self-management of chronic disease in primary care. *JAMA*. 2002 Nov; **288**(19): 2469–75.

41 Wasson JH, Bartels S. CARE Vital Signs supports patient-centered, collaborative care. *J Ambul Care Manage*. 2009 Jan–Mar; **32**(1): 56–71.

42 Geisinger Health System; 2010. Available at: www.geisinger.org/ (accessed March 19, 2010).

43 Barnes J, Nichols L, Weinberg M. *Grand Junction, Colorado: a health community that works*; 2009. Available at: www.medicalhistory.com/home/index.asp (accessed March 19, 2010).

44 Shea S, Hripcsak G. Accelerating the use of electronic health records in physician practices. *N Engl J Med*. 2010 Jan; **362**(3): 192–5.

45 Shachak A, Jadad AR. Electronic health records in the age of social networks and global telecommunications. *JAMA*. 2010 Feb; **303**(5): 452–3.

46 Adler KG. E-prescribing: why the fuss? *Fam Pract Manag*. 2009 Jan–Feb; **16**(1): 22–7.

47 Friedman MA, Schueth A, Bell DS. Interoperable electronic prescribing in the United States: a progress report. *Health Aff (Millwood)*. 2009 Mar–Apr; **28**(2): 393–403.

48 Cassel C. Keynote Address at the 10th Annual Summit on Redesigning the Clinical Office Practice, Vancouver, BC, Canada. March 23, 2009.

49 Grumbach K, Bodenheimer T, Grundy P. *The Outcomes of Implementing Patient-centered Medical Home Interventions: a review of the evidence on quality, access and costs from recent prospective evaluation studies*. Patient-centred Primary Care Collaborative; 2009 Aug: pp. 1–6.

50 Fisher E. *Rethinking Healthcare: insights from regional variations*. March 8, 2010. Leff B, Reider L, Frick KD, Scharfstein DO, Boyd CM, Frey K, *et al*. Guided care and the cost of complex healthcare: a preliminary report. *Am J Manag Care*. 2009 Aug; **15**(8): 555–9.

51 Leff B, Reider L, Frick KD, Scharfstein DO, Boyd CM, Frey K, *et al*. Guided care and the cost of complex healthcare: a preliminary report. *Am J Manag Care*. 2009 Aug; **15**(8): 555–9.

52 Patterson K, Grenny J, McMillan R, Switzler A. *Crucial Conversations: tools for talking when the stakes are high*. New York: McGraw-Hill; 2002.

53 Johns C. *Engaging Reflection in Practice: a narrative approach*. Oxford: Blackwell Publishing; 2006.

54 Engel JD, Zarconi J, Pethtel LL, Missimi SA. *Narrative in Health Care: healing patients, practitioners, profession, and community*. Oxford and New York: Radcliffe Publishing; 2008.

55 American Academy of Family Physicians. *Downcoding and Blending*; 2006. Available at: www.aafp.org/online/en/home/policy/privatesector/topics/payment/blending.html (accessed March 19, 2010).

56 Woolf SH. A closer look at the economic argument for disease prevention. *JAMA*. 2009 Feb; **301**(5): 536–8.

57 Wenger E, McDermott R, Snyder WM. *Cultivating Communities of Practice*. Cambridge, MA: Harvard Business Press; 2002.

58 Endsley S, Kirkegaard M, Linares A. Working together: communities of practice in family medicine. *Fam Pract Manage.* 2005; **12**(1): 28–32.

59 McGeeney T. The TransforMED project. *Am Fam Physician.* 2008 Mar; **77**(6): 751–2.

60 Crabtree BF, Nutting PA, Miller WL, Stange KC, Stewart EE, Jaén CR. Summary of the National Demonstration Project and recommendations for the patient-centered medical home. *Ann Fam Med.* 2010 May; 8(Suppl.): S80–90.

61 Makeham MA, Dovey SM, County M, Kidd MR. An international taxonomy for errors in general practice: a pilot study. *Med J Aust.* 2002 Jul; **177**(2): 68–72.

62 Rosser W, Dovey S, Bordman R, White D, Crighton E, Drummond N. Medical errors in primary care: results of an international study of family practice. *Can Fam Physician.* 2005 Mar; **51**: 386–7.

63 Kostopoulou O, Delaney BC, Munro CW. Diagnostic difficulty and error in primary care: a systematic review. *Fam Pract.* 2008 Dec; **25**(6): 400–13.

64 Solberg LI, Asche SE, Averbeck BM, Hayek AM, Schmitt KG, Lindquist TC, *et al.* Can patient safety be measured by surveys of patient experiences? *Jt Comm J Qual Patient Saf.* 2008 May; **34**(5): 266–74.

65 Fine M, Peters JW. *The Nature of Health: how America lost, and can regain, a basic human value.* Oxford: Radcliffe Publishing; 2007.

66 Rosenthal MP, Rabinowitz HK, Diamond JJ, Markham FW Jr. Medical students' specialty choice and the need for primary care. Our future. *Prim Care.* 1996 Mar; **23**(1): 155–67.

67 Senf JH, Campos-Outcalt D, Kutob R. Factors related to the choice of family medicine: a reassessment and literature review. *J Am Board Fam Pract.* 2003 Nov–Dec; **16**(6): 502–12.

68 Bodenheimer T. *Building Teams in Primary Care: lessons learned.* Oakland, CA: California Health Care Foundation; 2007.

69 Scholtes P, Joiner B, Streibel B. *The Team Handbook.* 3rd ed. Madison, WI: Oriel; 2003.

Afterword

It is too quiet for a morning. Hurriedly I stumble from exam room to room trying to keep up with my electronic medical record charting and wishing for the sunset and the end of another day at the practice assembly line. Jeannette, the medical receptionist, quietly clutches her coffee between methodically rooming patients and longing for sunset and meeting her friends at a local tavern. A patient, usually loquacious Anna, silently and sullenly puts on her coat preparing to leave unable to imagine a sunset. I told her the pain behind her ribs would go away. She, living inside the wisdom of her body, knew otherwise. Rushing toward the other end of the day, I stopped listening and opened space for medical error. We bumped in the hall as she left and our eyes met. I saw the silence; it felt like thunder. We return to the room and start over. If you are reading these words, I hope it means you just finished reading this remarkable book of hope by my friends, Tony Kuzel and John Engel. If you haven't started shaking up yourself and your practice, then start over. This book celebrates sunrise and wants action and vigorous conversations. Medical errors in primary care are personal, systemic, and relational. They were also too quiet until this book howled.

Improving the quality of primary care and the healers called into its service has been my own vocation for nearly 30 years. The patient stories that open this book painfully describe how challenging this work is. The overall situation in primary care is worse now, both for patients and clinicians, than 30 years ago, but, as refreshingly reviewed by Tony and John, dramatic possibilities and changes present themselves today. The American Academy of Family Physicians' National Demonstration Project of the PCMH, for which I was one of the evaluators, recently published its final results.[1] The messages are clear. (1) Highly motivated, independent practices can successfully implement many of the technical components of the PCMH and partially improve chronic illness care markers but at the risk of reducing patient-rated quality of care measures. (2) Delivery system and payment reform are essential to fully support primary care transformation. (3) Developing practices' internal capabilities is critical for successfully navigating the challenges of change and transformation and this may be the most important work for all of us until those system-level changes occur. So, don't put this book back on the shelf; you are holding a guide for building your practice's internal capability.

This book is a magical map for finding treasure in your practice. Follow the 10 steps. Somewhere between step two and step five, a twinkle appears, and between step eight and ten, an ever-expanding smile fills your face and a miracle can happen. You feel drawn to colleagues and patients. You return home with a bounce and excitement. The next morning dawns and you hear the old call and eagerly set off for the practice. What happened? The curve of generosity touched you by surprise from behind. Your new healing home is alive with voices and stories and has become a living library of growing wisdom. The answer is always "Yes" and everyone is awake. I have witnessed this miracle less than a handful of times over the past 30 years. What was special about the miracle practices? How could yours be one? Following the 10 steps gets you started, but the magic requires that you manifest three special aspects of leadership.

Leadership is engaging with self and others to make sense and find a way through life's mazes. It begins with finding a way into and out of self, the work of the reflective practitioner eloquently noted in the foreword by David Loxtercamp. Within every maze is a labyrinth—a way into and out of the confusions and despair. This labyrinth is a spiritual mobius strip where there is only one edge, where the inner and outer are the same—a hidden wholeness. Create labyrinths within your inner world; **practice a daily spiritual discipline**. Spiritual growth is alchemy; it converts distress into hopeful joy and generates a reservoir of love that overflows from within to without. Helping your practice and patients discover their own ways and labyrinths involves leading through storytelling, our uniquely human means of sense-making. **Practice narrative competence** as wonderfully demonstrated throughout this book. Does the office staff know your story? What are the practice stories? What would all of you and your patients like them to be? These are all stories from the more ancient oral tradition; thus, there is no final version. With healing and primary care, there is no end; the story always continues. Primary care is about sequels and daily acts of creative imagination. Keep re-telling and making sense.

Leadership is creating space and intention for better and crucial conversations. Physicians too often believe that leadership means giving directions and being the boss. That is one meaning, but in my experience it is also a guaranteed miracle killer. The leadership of transformation generates, encourages, supports, values, abides, and humbly appreciates power knowing that inspired action emerges without being forced. The key is making it safe for everyone because we are all vulnerable. This is work of developing internal capability through better conversations and focuses on strengthening core, building adaptive reserve, and enhancing attentiveness to the local environment. Your practice's core consists of its resources, organizational structure (i.e. leadership, compensation, reward, and accountability systems), and functional processes which include the clinical care, operations, and finance processes. The majority of the 10 steps suggested by Kuzel and Engel significantly enhance the core. The adaptive reserve refers to those aspects of your practice that assure success in times of major change. In times of stability and economic prosperity, these features aren't necessary to get by, but in times like now, they are essential. Adaptive reserve features include regular whole practice meetings with times for reflection, facilitative leadership, a repository of helpful stories about the practice, the ability to improvise, and a learning culture. Building adaptive reserve requires frequent communication and multiple conversations about what's really important. Can your medical assistant or nurse challenge your care plan? Can your receptionist address a patient's needs without your approval? Do all of you identify and discuss your mistakes at regular meetings? **Practice difficult conversations** every day.

Leadership is "standing by words"[2] with intentional integrity. Language is one of our most powerful tools for healing and for hurting. Choose words intentionally and respect them as you do your patients and each other. Standing by words requires the virtue and skills of surefootedness. Surefootedness is the secret of the wilderness walker, the tracker, the backcountry skier, and effective primary care leaders. It involves moving through the world from your center and not moving ahead of it like the typical Westerner. When having to move fast and with little control, staying centered is a very small sweet spot between panic and disaster. But it is a tiny, nearly invisible balancing point of infinite joy. It is the place of surefootedness, moving "just-in-time" while prepared for "just-in-case." Always begin the next step from that place, and you are as ready as possible for whatever surprise at whatever speed comes next.

PRACTICE SUREFOOTEDNESS

Let me share two examples of where we did not stand by our words with intentional integrity and contributed to primary care's sorry state. In the early 1990s, we unwisely accepted being called, "gatekeepers." We forgot our foundational mission of hospitality and being the place of an always open gate. Fortunately, our patients called us out. We are "hosts" offering hospitality to all whose bodies have betrayed them or fear they might. Not long after, many began calling us "providers" and now I continually hear my colleagues using the same word as self-reference. In the spirit of the cross-disciplinary team, I applaud the effort to find a word that embraced all the members of the clinical team, but why accept a word from the land of commoditization and sales? Insurance companies provide; primary care practice teams, the "clinicians," offer healing relationships that support and facilitate patients' healthy return into the emerging stories of their lives.

The advice in this book will certainly make you happier and your practice better but not yet into the promised land. Arriving there demands focused advocacy in partnership with our patients for delivery and payment reform. In the meantime, prepare and create the better future. Gut the old primary care house. Collaborate more; reach out and take more in while preserving and defending the ancient healing relationships. Our patients plead for more agency and greater communion. This is what is offered in this book for patients and practices and clinicians. We are each given agency in our own practice story again. Communion will not be far behind. We, as healers, are boundary walkers and keepers, edge walkers. We help people "come back," we assist them in "crossing over," and we reassure some they aren't really "at the boundary." Are we practicing boundary craft? Are we helping each other to live well, to thrive on the edge, to build our nests in storms, to hurl starfish back into the waves, to see the beauty and wholeness within and beyond brokenness?

Winds howling change are rushing out of the west moving thick cloud rivers across the sky and rustling every timber in our practices. Sit still, re-read this book and listen to the sounds of tempestuous movement. Waves of air sweep across the land. They break onto the evergreen boughs tossing them hither and yon in a restless dance of anticipation. They whistle through every small crack in your office. This is the weather of transition, of potential dramatic transformation. It is the burst of energy that fuels our awakening. The role of the healer is to facilitate change to greater wholeness. The role of the teacher is to prepare one for the changes. Tony and John are our teachers. I can't wait for the sunrise! How about you?

William L Miller, MD, MA
Allentown, Pennsylvania

REFERENCES

1 Crabtree BF, Nutting PA, Miller WL, Stange KC, Stewart EE, Jaén CR. Summary of the National Demonstration Project and recommendations for the patient-centered medical home. *Ann Fam Med.* 2010 May; 8(Suppl.): S80–90.
2 Berry W. *Standing by Words: essays.* San Francisco, CA: North Point Press; 1983.

Readers' theater

COMPOSITE OF FINDINGS FROM KUZEL, WOOLF, GILCHRIST ET AL. STUDY OF PATIENT REPORTS.[1]

Problems in primary care: a reader's theater vignette

Written by Anton J Kuzel, MD, MHPE, and first performed as part of a symposium on humanistic perspectives on medical error held by the Institute for Professionalism Inquiry in Akron, Ohio in March, 2005.[2]

Players: NARRATOR, PHONE TREE, PATIENT (African-American woman), RECEPTIONIST, NURSE and DOCTOR (female) *(Also four people named later who are called back by the nurse before the patient is called back could also be on stage, and leave one by one as their names are called.)*

Stage setup: NARRATOR'S chair off to one side; chairs for PHONE TREE, PATIENT, RECEPTIONIST, and DOCTOR arranged in a semicircle center stage; people who are called by the Nurse about midway through the performance can be in a line behind the semicircle, and they can come on stage and sit down when PATIENT returns to the stage; otherwise all players are present and seated at the start of the performance; players read their parts from the script and do not look at one another, nor at audience members.

NARRATOR:	What follows is a fictional experience that a patient has with trying to access her PCPs for an acute illness. The elements are based on a series of interviews that researchers in Ohio and Virginia conducted with primary care patients about problems with their primary health care that resulted in some harm to them, whether physical or psychological. The setting for the play is an urban area in Ohio, but what happens can and does happen in suburban and rural

communities in Ohio and Virginia, and, we suspect, in all 50 States.

PATIENT: (*Miming dialing a phone number, and muttering under her breath.*) Time for my phone tree experience.

PHONE TREE: Thank you for calling PrimeCare. If this is a medical emergency, hang up and dial 911. Our office hours are 9 a.m.–5 p.m., Monday through Friday. If you are calling after hours and need to speak to a physician, please call 555–0666 to have the answering service page the physician on call. If you are calling during regular business hours and have reached this message, please select from the following menu: If you want to schedule an appointment, please press 1. If you want to . . . (*fades*).

PATIENT: (*Sighing audibly, mimes pressing a key on phone.*)

PHONE TREE: Thank you. All receptionists are currently assisting other patients. Please stay on the line and your call will be answered in the order in which it was received. Did you know that PrimeCare doctors believe in personalized, preventive health care? Ask your doctor about what preventive services are right for you. Did you know that . . . (*fades*).

PATIENT: (*Mimes looking at watch.*)
If I hang up now, I might as well forget about seeing the doctor.

RECEPTIONIST: PrimeCare.

PATIENT: Yes, this is Latasha Robinson. I need to see Dr Farmer today. I'm sick.

RECEPTIONIST: I'm sorry, Ms Robinson, but Dr Farmer is fully booked today. The next available appointment is next Tuesday.

PATIENT: Look, I've been on hold listening to your ads for personalized health care for the past half hour. Either I need to see the doctor today, or you need to have her call me back as soon as possible.

RECEPTIONIST: I can leave a message for the doctor to call you, Ms Robinson. What is your number?

PATIENT: 555–1780. Will you give Dr Farmer the message right away? Don't you want to know what to tell her?

RECEPTIONIST: I will give Dr Farmer the message. I have a lot of other callers waiting, Ms Robinson. Good bye.

(PATIENT *gets up from her chair and walks off stage.* RECEPTIONIST *stands and faces away from audience briefly, then sits down again.* PATIENT *returns to the stage and approaches her former seat, but remains standing.*)

RECEPTIONIST:	(*Miming holding a telephone to her ear.*) Hold please. Yes, can I help you?
PATIENT:	I'm Latasha Robinson. I called yesterday and asked you to leave a message for Dr Farmer. I never got a call back. I need to see her today.
RECEPTIONIST:	Do you have an appointment?
PATIENT:	I don't think I would have gotten one if I tried. I talked to you yesterday and asked you to leave a message for Dr Farmer to call me as soon as possible, and I never got a call back. I am sick and I needed to be seen yesterday. I am here today, and I need to be seen by the doctor.
RECEPTIONIST:	Doctor is already overbooked for today. I will need to check with the nurse to see if we can fit you in. Please have a seat and I will call you up after I take care of the people on hold.
PATIENT:	(*Slumps into chair, shoulders sagging and head down; mimes looking at watch.*)
RECEPTIONIST:	Ms Robinson?
PATIENT:	(*Straightening up.*) Yes?
RECEPTIONIST:	I need to confirm your contact information and insurance. Please fill out the information sheet and give it back to me when you are done, along with your insurance card.
PATIENT:	I don't see why I need to do this every time I come here. Nothing has changed since my last visit.
RECEPTIONIST:	I'm sorry, Ms Robinson—it's office policy.
PATIENT:	(*Frustration in her voice.*) Seems to me your policies are all about *you*.
RECEPTIONIST:	(*No reply; mimes receiving a clipboard.*) The nurse will call you back. We have added you on to the doctor's schedule, but she was already overbooked. She will get to you as soon as she can.
PATIENT:	(*Shoulders slump and head bows, again; looks at watch.*)
NURSE:	Dr Zarconi? (*Pause.*) Dr Engel? (*Pause.*) Ms Missimi? (*Laughs.*) Did you know your name sounds kinda like Mississippi when I say it like that—Ms Missimi? (*Laughs again; pause.*) Ms Pethtel? (*Longer pause.*) Latasha Robinson?

PATIENT:	(*Straightening up.*) Here—coming.
NURSE:	Please follow me. Let's check your weight. Okay. You will be in room 6. Let's check your blood pressure. Okay. Now what seems to be the problem?
PATIENT:	I am sick. Been getting sicker for the past week. I tried to talk with Dr Farmer about it yesterday, but she never called me back. I have a terrific headache that's getting worse, and I don't get headaches. Nothing I've tried works for it. It's always there, and it keeps me from sleeping. I'm worried there is something seriously wrong, because I just don't get headaches.
NURSE:	Alright. I will let Dr Farmer know. She will be in to see you when she can—there are several other patients ahead of you. Change into this gown so you will be ready when she gets to you.
PATIENT:	(*Mimes changing into gown; mimes looking at watch; finally looks up.*)
DOCTOR:	Ms Jones, what seems to be the problem today?
PATIENT:	I'm not Ms Jones. I'm Latasha Robinson.
DOCTOR	They gave me the wrong chart. Oh well, I'll do the best I can without your chart. So you have a headache.
PATIENT:	Yes, I explained to the nurse—(*Get's cut off.*)
DOCTOR:	Yes, I know—she told me. Look, it's probably nothing serious. Your blood pressure is fine. Let me do a brief neurological exam on you. Follow my finger with your eyes. Stick out your tongue. Show me your teeth. Hold your arms out and don't let me push them down. Touch your finger with your nose. Now touch my finger. Now do that with the other hand. Push your left leg out against my hand. Do that with the other leg. Stand up and put your feet together. Close your eyes. Open your eyes. Walk to the door and back. It looks like there is nothing serious going on here. I'm going to give you something for pain. Call me if you have any more problems. (*Mimes writing prescription.*)
PATIENT:	But I'm still worried there is something wrong. You don't even have the right chart to look at.
DOCTOR:	Sorry about that, but you look like you've been basically healthy, so I'm sure this is nothing serious. Here's the pre-scription. I've got to run now—they added you on to my

PATIENT:

schedule, and I was already overbooked. Call me if you have any more problems. (*Gets up from chair and walks off stage.*)

(*Mouth open—says nothing for a few seconds.*)

And I waited two hours for *that*? And all those *white* folks getting called back first, and some of them *doctors*. And wasn't that nurse having a *good* time with that Mississippi lady? And the wrong chart, and they don't even care about that. I am *not* coming back here again. I might as well go to the emergency room and wait eight hours—I bet I would still get better service than I get here.

NARRATOR:

Some of you may have already guessed this, but the doctor's name for this play was not a random choice. In the original study, when the investigators asked one of the respondents how she would characterize her relationship with her PCPs, she replied, Well, I guess like farmer–cow.

REFERENCES

1 Kuzel AJ, Woolf SH, Gilchrist VJ, Engel JD, LaVeist TA, Vincent C, *et al*. Patient reports of preventable problems and harms in primary health care. *Ann Fam Med*. 2004 Jul–Aug; 2(4): 333–40.

2 Kuzel AJ. Problems in primary care: a readers' theater vignette. Presentation to Institute for Professionalism Inquiry, Akron, OH. March, 2005.

HowsYourHealth survey

PATIENT SURVEY: PATIENT-REPORTED MEASURES TO ASSESS OFFICE PRACTICE QUALITY OF CARE

This survey is given to patients aged 50–69 years. The survey questions are derived from items in the HowsYourHealth.org web-based survey. Because survey responses involve entry into a file for scoring, many practices find it advantageous to offer the web-based version for free, which can be obtained by registering at www.IdealMedicalHome.org.

We are asking some of our patients, aged 50–69, to complete a brief survey about their health and health care. We are using this information to improve our services.

We do not wish for any patient names. Thank you very much.

Please check with a tick (✓) the best answers. After completing the survey, place it in the self-addressed stamped envelope.

1 During the past four weeks, have you been bothered often or always by emotional problems such as feeling anxious, depressed, irritable, sad or downhearted, and blue?

___ Not at all (1)

___ Slightly (2)

___ Moderately (3)

___ Quite a bit (4)

___ Extremely (5)

If you checked this, is your doctor or nurse aware of the problem?

___ Yes (1) ___ No (2) ___ I am not sure (3)

2 During the past four weeks, how much body pain have you generally had?

___ No pain (1)

___ Very mild pain (2)

___ Mild pain (3)

___ Moderate pain (4)
___ Severe pain (5)
If you checked this, is your doctor or nurse aware of the problem?
___ Yes (1) ___ No (2) ___ I am not sure (3)

3 Has a doctor told you that you have any of these problems?
   Please check (✓) all that applies.
   ___ High blood pressure (1)
   ___ Heart trouble or hardening of the arteries (2)
   ___ Diabetes (sugar) (3)
   ___ Arthritis (4)
   ___ Asthma, bronchitis, or emphysema (5)
   ___ Serious obesity (more than 15% overweight) (6)
   If you checked (✓) that you have high blood pressure, heart trouble,
   diabetes, arthritis, breathing problems, or obesity, *please answer questions
   4–8. If not, go to question 9.*

4 In general, how would you rate the information given to you about these
   problem(s) by your doctor or a nurse? Please check (✓) the best answer.
   ___ Excellent (1)
   ___ Very good (2)
   ___ Good (3)
   ___ Fair (4)
   ___ Poor (5)
   ___ I do not remember receiving any information (6)

5 If you indicated that you have breathing problems:
   How would you rate the information your doctor or a nurse gave you
   about how to adjust medicines for your shortness of breath?
   ___ Excellent (1)
   ___ Very good (2)
   ___ Good (3)
   ___ Fair (4)
   ___ Poor (5)
   ___ I do not remember receiving any information (6)

6 If you indicated that you have diabetes:
   How often do you keep your blood glucose (sugar) within normal range
   (between 80 and 150)?

___ I do not test my blood glucose (1)
___ All the time (2)
___ Often (3)
___ Sometimes (4)
___ Rarely (5)
___ Never (6)

7 If you have high blood pressure:
   Do you check your own blood pressure?
   ___ Yes, often (1) ___ Yes, sometimes (2) ___ Almost never (3)
   ___ Never (4)

8 What was your last blood pressure? What was the high number of your
   blood pressure (systolic blood pressure)?
   ___ Under 100 (1)
   ___ 100–120 (2)
   ___ 121–130 (3)
   ___ 131–140 (4)
   ___ 141–150 (5)
   ___ 151–160 (6)
   ___ 161–170 (7)
   ___ Higher than 171 (8)
   ___ I do not know (9)

9 Do you have one person you think of as your personal doctor or nurse?
   ___ Yes (1) ___ No (2)

10 How easy is it for you to get medical care when you need it?
    ___ Very easy (1)
    ___ Easy (2)
    ___ Somewhat difficult (3)
    ___ Very difficult (4)
    ___ I have not needed medical care (5)

11 When you visit your doctor's office, how often is it well organized and
    efficient and does not waste your time?
    ___ Most of the time (1)
    ___ Some of the time (2)

___ Almost never is it efficient. It often wastes my time (3)
___ Does not apply to me. I seldom visit a doctor's office (4)

12 How confident are you that you can control and manage most of your health problems?
___ Very confident (1)
___ Somewhat confident (2)
___ Not very confident (3)
___ I do not have any health problems (4)

13 Are there things about your medical care that could be better?
___ No, my care is perfect (1)
___ Yes, some things (2)
___ Yes, a lot of things (3)

14 Do you have enough money to buy the things that you need to live everyday, such as food, clothing, or housing?
___ Yes, always (1)
___ Sometimes (2)
___ No (3)

15 In the past two years, have you had a test for cancer of the bowel?
___ Yes (1) ___ No (2) ___ No, but I have had a colonoscopy in the past nine years (3)

16 Do you think that any of your medications are making you sick?
___ Yes (1)
___ No (2)
___ Maybe, I am not sure (3)
___ I am not taking any medications (4)

17 In the *past year*, have you been in the hospital or visited an emergency department?
___ Yes (1) ___ No (2)

18 In the *past three months*, did you have an illness or injury that kept you in bed for all or most of the day?
___ Yes (1) ___ No (2)

19 During the *past two weeks*, how much did physical health or emotional problems keep you from working the hours you needed to work?
___ Physical or emotional problems *did not limit* my ability to work at all (1)
___ Physical or emotional problems *did limit* my ability to work a small amount (about 10%–20%) (2)
___ Physical or emotional problems *did limit* my ability to work a large amount (more than 20%) (3)

20 When you think about your health care, how much do you agree or disagree with this statement:
"I receive exactly what I want and need exactly when and how I want and need it."
___ I agree strongly (1)___ I somewhat agree (2)
___ I somewhat disagree (3) ___ I disagree strongly (4)

21 Are you seeing a specialist physician?
___ Yes (1) ___ No (2) ___ I am not sure (3)
If you answered *Yes*, please continue to Question 22.

22 If you are seeing a specialist physician and your primary physician, do you have one doctor who you feel is in charge of your medical care?
___ Yes (1) ___ No (2) ___ I am not sure (3)

Thank you for completing this survey!

Please return in the enclosed self-addressed stamped envelope.

Index

Entries in **bold** refer to boxes, tables and figures.

preventive services 9, 54, 57, 63, 69, 86, 92–3, 104
primary care
  ambulatory 8–9
  evaluating **60**, 61
  financing of 68–70
  ideal model of 63
  new rules for **71–2**
  problems of **59**
  reasons for poor outcomes in 72
  shift away from xiv, 6
  shifting towards 103–4
  success stories in 63–4, 66–7, 69–71
  tasks of 8, 54
psychological harms 4, 20

quality improvement 3, 55–6, 70, 72–4

racism 3, 20
rapid access scheduling 65, 89–92
rationality, technical ix, xi
receptionists 33–4, 40, 43–4, 86
referrals 4, **16**, 26–7, 35, 42, 74
reflective practitioners vii, ix–x, xiii, 112
reimbursement rates 104
relationship breakdown 11, 17–18
relationship-centered care (RCC) xv, 8, 77–8
reliability 72–3

Schon, Donald ix
self-actualization xv
self-treatment 73
services, basket of 54, 63
shots 32, 43–4
spirituality 112
surefootedness 113
survey tools 4, 68, 120–4

team care 69–70, 74, 86–8, 93, 97, 106
technical errors 2, 5, 11, 17, 106
test results
  following up on 5
  getting 30–1, 64
  miscommunication of 4, 18
  responding to 73
three Ts **96–7**
To Err is Human 1, 3, 8
transparency xii, 71
triple aim 8, 53

urgi-centers 89, 94
urinary tract infections 30–2

Virginia Academy of Family Physicians (VAFP) 105
voicemail 15, 42

X-rays 13, 41, 48